Leveraging GenAI for Machine Learning Education in Public Health

Ricky Leung

Leveraging GenAI for Machine Learning Education in Public Health

ChatGPT and R

Springer

Ricky Leung
School of Public Health, Division of Social and Behavioral Sciences
University of Memphis
Memphis, TN, USA

ISBN 978-3-032-08676-1 ISBN 978-3-032-08677-8 (eBook)
https://doi.org/10.1007/978-3-032-08677-8

This Springer imprint is published by the registered company Springer Nature Switzerland AG
The registered company address is: Gewerbestrasse 11, 6330 Cham, Switzerland

Preface

This book is written for public health faculty, students, and practitioners who wish to learn machine learning programming through the guided use of ChatGPT, one of today's most widely used generative AI tools. It is designed as a practical companion rather than a script to be followed line by line. Because ChatGPT is a large language model, its outputs—such as R code—may vary slightly across sessions and versions. Readers should treat the prompts, examples, and exercises as a structured guide, while still validating results and documenting assumptions. The aim is to offer a clear bridge as our field moves into an AI-enabled era.

Public health work increasingly relies on computational methods for surveillance, evaluation, and decision support. Generative AI lowers barriers to entry, but responsible use still demands statistical reasoning and domain expertise. Each chapter pairs ChatGPT-assisted coding with core analytic concepts, emphasizing transparency, version control, and simple safeguards that help teams adopt these tools responsibly. More advanced approaches—such as agentic AI systems that plan tasks and call external tools—will reshape how we teach and conduct analytic work; those topics deserve a dedicated volume. Here, the emphasis is immediate: learning by doing, with clear prompts, vetted code, and plain guidance.

This project was sustained by several professional milestones. During the writing, I began establishing the AI for Health Research Lab at the University of Memphis with support from an NIH grant. I also led and participated in a number of new AI initiatives at the University of Memphis and served as an external advisor to other institutes and funding agencies. Lab members provided steady help and protected time, which made completion possible. I also thank colleagues at Memphis—Ashish Joshi, Dipankar Dasgupta, Satish Kedia, Marian Levy, Ilias Kavouras, Arunava Roy, Rameshwari Prasad, Joomi Kim, and Sharon Griffin—for their encouragement and collaboration.

My interest in high-tech science grew under my advisor, Joan Fujimura. I also benefitted from Kjell Doksum, whose guidance sharpened both quantitative reasoning and scientific interpretation. The initial idea for this book crystallized during a sabbatical supported by the University at Albany. I thank colleagues there—Wendy

Weller, Yuchi Young, Julia Hastings, Diane Dewar, and Shao Lin—for covering teaching and research while I spent time at the National University of Singapore (NUS) and the Chinese University of Hong Kong (CUHK). I am especially grateful to Andy Rose, Sam Yam, and Michelle Loke at NUS, and to Tony Tam and C. Y. Chiu at CUHK. I also had the privilege of mentoring many brilliant students across these institutions.

This book is dedicated to my mother, Bing Yee Tse, whose endless encouragement and loving care shaped my path. During a difficult time for our family, my brother Howard Leung and many relatives provided deep support; I thank them enormously. Finally, my heartfelt thanks go to my wife, Jing Li, and to our children, Arthur and Hugh Leung, for their constant support—and for offering the most upfront and helpful criticism of my work.

I hope this volume serves as a practical starting point for public health professionals who wish to use generative AI to learn, prototype, and communicate machine learning methods with rigor and humility.

Hartsdale, NY, USA
August 15, 2025

Ricky Leung

Competing Interests The author has no competing interests to declare that are relevant to the content of this manuscript.

Contents

About the Author

Ricky Leung is Professor and Director of Social and Behavioral Sciences at the University of Memphis School of Public Health in Tennessee, USA. A leading scholar at the intersection of artificial intelligence, machine learning, public health and management, he has published extensively on AI and other emerging technologies in high-impact journals such as *Lancet*, *JAMA*, and *Organization Science*. His research has received support from NSF, CDC, NIH, and other public agencies and private organizations, and he has also served as a panelist for some of these organizations. As an educator, he teaches courses in relation to AI, Health and Society, Responsible AI in Public Health, AI and Talent Management, and GenAI-assisted Machine Learning Programming, equipping future professionals with the skills to navigate the evolving AI landscape. He previously served as the Interim Director of the Global Center for AI in Mental Health at the University at Albany and is currently establishing an NIH-sponsored AI for Health Lab, and a new Center on Responsible AI in Public Health at the University of Memphis.

Part I
Laying the Foundation

Chapter 1
Introduction

Learning Objectives
By the end of this chapter, readers will be able to:

1. **Explain** how artificial intelligence (AI) and machine learning (ML) can help solve public health challenges.
2. **Name** major ML techniques and their relevance in public health data.
3. **Discuss** ethical issues and risks in AI-based public health research.
4. **Assess** pros and cons of using GenAI tools like ChatGPT in learning.
5. **Describe** the book's structure and its role in building public health data skills.

Background

The emergence of large language models (LLMs) and generative AI (GenAI) tools—such as ChatGPT, Claude, Gemini, and Copilot—has reshaped how individuals learn and interact with complex technologies. These tools offer a novel learning pathway by assisting users in generating code, interpreting machine learning (ML) outputs, and troubleshooting programming errors. In doing so, GenAI bridges abstract AI concepts with the concrete skill of programming, allowing learners to engage with ML in a more intuitive and iterative manner. LLMs have already demonstrated notable capabilities, such as passing medical licensing examinations and enabling personalized learning strategies (Kung et al., 2023).

Despite these advances, AI remains vague or inaccessible to many public health professionals. Questions such as "Can AI do everything for us?", "What exactly does it cover?", and "How can we use AI responsibly?" reflect this uncertainty. This book addresses these concerns by positioning machine learning programming—

Supplementary Information The online version contains supplementary material available at https://doi.org/10.1007/978-3-032-08677-8_1.

R. Leung, *Leveraging GenAI for Machine Learning Education in Public Health*,
https://doi.org/10.1007/978-3-032-08677-8_1

specifically using the R language—as an entry point for understanding and applying AI in public health contexts. Rather than treating AI as a black box, this approach emphasizes hands-on coding, model evaluation, and interpretability. These competencies are essential for public health professionals, especially those with backgrounds in epidemiology, biostatistics, or policy analysis, who may not have formal training in software development or algorithm design (Hamilton et al., 2021).

At the same time, GenAI presents risks. It can produce hallucinated outputs, reinforce existing biases, or misrepresent technical concepts. Therefore, responsible use requires the very competencies it seeks to support: foundational knowledge of ML methods (e.g., supervised and unsupervised learning) and awareness of ethical risks such as privacy concerns, transparency, and fairness in model outcomes (Dwivedi et al., 2023).

This book is built around that premise. While GenAI can streamline code generation, model interpretation, and iterative refinement, effective use still depends on a solid grounding in ML concepts. Public health professionals must acquire basic programming skills to evaluate, refine, and validate GenAI-generated content. Without such skills, users may fail to detect hallucinations, misapplied techniques, or biased algorithms that exacerbate health inequities. R programming—the core language used throughout this book—provides a technical foundation for running, assessing, and adjusting ML models. By combining the accessibility of GenAI with practical training in R, learners will be better prepared to apply AI responsibly and effectively in public health domains.

Public health professionals often engage with different aspects of data and decision-making. This book offers a broadly applicable resource because AI—often perceived as an abstract or futuristic concept—is grounded in specific tools and techniques, particularly machine learning. The increasing availability of large-scale data in healthcare has made ML methods highly relevant for addressing real-world challenges (Obermeyer & Emanuel, 2016; Topol, 2019). ML enables researchers to analyze vast datasets, detect risk patterns, forecast health outcomes, and guide decisions in areas such as disease surveillance, health behavior, and service delivery. Even more promising is the opportunity to use GenAI as a learning tool to explore this domain—specifically, to master ML programming through guided, interactive practice.

Why Learning a Programming Language Still Matters—and Why R

Here is a key puzzle for many public health professionals: If GenAI tools can generate code and explain technical concepts, why should they invest time in learning programming languages like R? The answer centers on the need for technical literacy—both to responsibly evaluate AI-generated solutions and to learn through active engagement. While GenAI can assist with coding and provide step-by-step explanations, its outputs are only as reliable as the user's ability to critically assess and adapt them.

Even in an AI-assisted environment, foundational programming knowledge remains essential. GenAI tools can generate plausible-looking code and explanations, but they are prone to hallucinations and errors. As documented in recent studies, LLMs often produce non-functional code or logical inconsistencies that may not raise obvious flags but can result in silent failures (Bang et al., 2023). In public health, where decisions drawn from analytic outputs may shape interventions or inform policy, such errors can have serious consequences.

Empirical research and classroom observations further suggest that students who rely heavily on GenAI without understanding core programming concepts often encounter difficulties adapting or debugging code in novel situations. Users tend to overestimate the reliability of AI-generated content, especially when outputs are incomplete or subtly incorrect (Vaithilingam et al., 2022). This reflects a broader principle: using GenAI effectively depends on the very knowledge it seeks to simplify. Without a basic understanding of programming, public health professionals may not be equipped to judge whether a machine learning model is appropriate for their data, population, or ethical context.

Among available tools, R stands out as particularly suited to public health applications and machine learning implementation. Originally designed for statistical computing and data visualization, R supports reproducible research—an important goal for health professionals working with complex, population-level datasets. Its open-source nature and rich ecosystem of packages for epidemiology, spatial data, and machine learning offer a cost-effective and adaptable platform for diverse analytic tasks.

The RStudio integrated development environment further enhances accessibility, with user-friendly features such as syntax highlighting, version control integration, and interactive data visualization. Its notebook-style interface encourages reproducible workflows that are central to rigorous public health practice (Peng, 2020). These attributes make R a practical and scalable option for those new to programming.

ChatGPT as a Learning Assistant: Benefits, Limitations, and the Need for Critical Oversight

Building on the case for foundational programming literacy, this section examines how public health professionals can effectively incorporate generative AI tools—specifically ChatGPT—into their learning process. While these tools offer unique opportunities to support the acquisition of R programming and machine learning (ML) skills, their use must be guided by critical oversight and informed judgment.

ChatGPT functions as an accessible and responsive learning assistant. It can explain statistical concepts, generate R code snippets, debug programming errors, and deconstruct complex ML workflows into manageable steps. Its interactive format allows learners to engage in an iterative dialogue: asking clarification questions, exploring multiple approaches, and receiving immediate feedback. For public health professionals new to coding, these features can reduce barriers to entry and accelerate skill development.

However, these advantages must be tempered by a clear understanding of the tool's limitations. ChatGPT can generate text that is syntactically correct and stylistically polished, yet factually incorrect or technically flawed. In programming contexts, it may suggest outdated functions, misapply statistical methods, or produce non-functional or subtly erroneous code. These so-called "hallucinations"are especially risky for novice users, who may not yet possess the conceptual grounding needed to detect errors (Alkaissi & McFarlane, 2023).

Throughout this book, I emphasize that ChatGPT's output should never be accepted uncritically. Its responses are based on probabilistic associations rather than genuine comprehension. While this does not render the tool useless, it necessitates a mindset of verification. Empirical research has documented high rates of inaccuracies in AI-generated technical content, including fabricated references and misleading recommendations (Sallam, 2023). Accordingly, each output from ChatGPT—whether a line of code or a statistical explanation—must be scrutinized, tested, and cross-checked against authoritative documentation and established practice.

To use ChatGPT effectively, learners must cultivate both programming and evaluative competencies. This includes crafting precise prompts that define the intended use case, specifying R version or package dependencies, and contextualizing questions within appropriate methodological frameworks. All code generated should be tested in isolated environments before application to real-world datasets. In addition, learners should triangulate ChatGPT's suggestions with textbooks, peer-reviewed articles, and official package documentation. Without these safeguards, users may inadvertently introduce flawed methods into their analyses—undermining research quality and, potentially, public health decision-making (Vaithilingam et al., 2022; Kazemitabaar et al., 2024).

Nonetheless, when approached with care, ChatGPT offers valuable pedagogical support. It can illustrate alternative coding strategies, recommend debugging techniques, and present diverse solutions that foster deeper understanding. Its interactivity also supports exploratory learning, allowing users to test ideas in real time and refine their reasoning. For educators, ChatGPT can serve as a supplementary resource, helping to develop practice exercises, simulate data scenarios, and provide tailored explanations suited to different learning styles.

The key to successful use of ChatGPT in ML education is maintaining a careful balance between leveraging its capabilities and exercising critical oversight. This is particularly important in public health, where the consequences of analytical errors extend beyond individual projects to broader population outcomes. Learners must view ChatGPT as a tool for exploration—one that enhances, rather than replaces, foundational knowledge and domain-specific expertise.

This balanced perspective—integrating the efficiency of AI with the rigor of traditional programming education—underpins the pedagogical approach of this book. The next section outlines how these principles are operationalized through the structure of the text, offering a roadmap for learning R programming and ML with ChatGPT as a thoughtfully integrated assistant.

Purpose of the Book

This book is written for public health students and professionals who seek a practical, accessible introduction to machine learning (ML) models with direct relevance to applied public health practice. It presents a broad spectrum of essential techniques, beginning with core supervised learning models—such as logistic regression, decision trees, and random forests—and extending to unsupervised methods including k-means clustering, hierarchical clustering, and principal component analysis. More advanced approaches such as support vector machine, gradient boosting, deep learning, and natural language processing for unstructured health data are also introduced. Each method is demonstrated using both built-in R datasets and realistic simulated datasets created by the author, illustrating scenarios such as predicting disease outbreaks, optimizing resource allocation, and analyzing patient feedback.

As emphasized in previous sections, programming knowledge remains critical for using AI tools responsibly. Accordingly, this book positions R programming not only as a technical skill, but also as a foundation for developing evaluative judgment. Structured exercises, case-based projects, and guided code walkthroughs are included throughout the text to ensure hands-on experience. Learners are guided through the full process of using R and RStudio to clean, analyze, and model health data; apply appropriate ML techniques to real-world public health challenges; and interpret model results with a focus on accuracy, transparency, and explainability.

At the same time, this book reflects the growing role of generative AI tools like ChatGPT in public health education. Rather than discouraging their use, the book demonstrates how to integrate these tools as learning companions—offering support in coding, explanation, and debugging—while maintaining a rigorous stance on their limitations. Readers will learn how to craft prompts, test outputs, and evaluate the reliability of GenAI assistance in the context of applied ML tasks. Throughout, the emphasis remains on critical oversight, responsible application, and alignment with public health values.

Ultimately, this book aims to cultivate both technical competencies and reflective practice. By learning to work with R, applying machine learning methods to realistic problems, and using GenAI tools with discernment, readers will be prepared to engage with AI technologies in ways that are not only effective but also ethically and contextually appropriate for public health work.

Book and Chapter Overview

This book is organized into three main sections, each building upon the last to equip readers with the skills, tools, and critical thinking needed to apply machine learning (ML) and generative AI (GenAI) in public health responsibly and effectively. The structure follows a progressive learning path—from foundational concepts to practical implementation and finally to ethical and professional considerations.

Part I: Laying the Foundation

This opening section introduces essential concepts and tools, serving as a starting point for readers who may have limited programming experience. It also reinforces the importance of maintaining programming literacy, even in an era where GenAI tools are increasingly accessible.

Chapter 1: Introduction

Provides an overview of the book, emphasizing the growing importance of AI and ML in public health. It introduces major trends, typical applications, and key learning outcomes.

Chapter 2: Understanding AI and Machine Learning for Public Health

Presents core ML concepts—such as supervised, unsupervised, and deep learning—using accessible explanations and relevant public health examples. The chapter also explains how data science enhances traditional areas like epidemiology and biostatistics.

Chapter 3: Getting Started with ChatGPT and RStudio

Guides readers through the setup of R and RStudio and introduces ChatGPT as a supportive learning assistant. The chapter emphasizes prompt design, validation of AI-generated output, and responsible use. Readers practice writing basic R scripts while learning how to use ChatGPT to explain, generate, and debug code.

Part II: Machine Learning Techniques and Applications

This section focuses on applying key ML techniques to address real-world public health problems. It moves from foundational models to more advanced approaches, with all techniques demonstrated using both R's built-in datasets and simulated public health scenarios.

Chapter 4: Supervised Learning I—Classification

Covers classification models including K-nearest neighbors (KNN), logistic regression, decision trees, and random forests. Applications include predicting disease risk and modeling health service utilization patterns.

Chapter 5: Supervised Learning II—Regression
Introduces regression models such as linear regression, polynomial regression, ridge regression, and lasso regression. Readers apply these models to forecast continuous outcomes like disease burden, healthcare costs, and population health indicators.

Chapter 6: Unsupervised Learning
Explores clustering and dimensionality reduction methods, including k-means clustering, hierarchical clustering, and principal component analysis. Case studies include patient segmentation and analysis of health behavior patterns.

Chapter 7: Advanced Models and Natural Language Processing
Presents advanced ML techniques such as support vector machines, gradient boosting, and deep learning. The chapter also introduces natural language processing (NLP) for analyzing unstructured health data—including patient narratives, clinical notes, and social media—using methods like tokenization, sentiment analysis, and topic modeling.

Part III: Ethical, Responsible, and Real-World AI Applications

The final section focuses on real-world implementation, ethical implications, and model interpretability—key considerations for responsible use of AI in public health settings.

Chapter 8: Real-World Applications of Supervised Learning
Features comprehensive case studies that integrate multiple ML techniques. Topics include optimizing vaccine distribution, developing outbreak forecasting systems, and designing health communication interventions. Each project guides the reader through the full ML pipeline, from data preparation to evaluation.

Chapter 9: Explainability and Reproducibility in ML
Addresses the importance of interpretability in health-related machine learning. It covers techniques for model explanation, feature importance analysis, and strategies for communicating results to policymakers, clinicians, and community partners.

Chapter 10: Future Directions and Continuous Learning in AI
Explores topics such as data privacy, algorithmic bias, transparency, and AI governance frameworks. It underscores the importance of lifelong learning, adapting to emerging technologies, and cultivating AI literacy as part of public health workforce development.

As you embark on this learning journey, remember that mastering machine learning for public health does not require becoming a computer scientist. Rather, it involves developing practical skills that can directly enhance your ability to address real-world health challenges. The combination of R programming and thoughtful use of AI tools like ChatGPT offers a powerful way to accelerate your learning while deepening conceptual understanding.

Whether you're writing your first R script, implementing a new ML algorithm, or interpreting complex model outputs, ChatGPT can serve as a supportive guide—helping you clarify ideas, troubleshoot problems, and explore alternative approaches. The chapters ahead will lead you step by step through this process, not only teaching what to do, but also how to think critically about AI-assisted learning. By the end of this book, you will have both the technical confidence and ethical awareness to apply machine learning and AI tools effectively in public health contexts. Let us begin this journey together.

Discussion Questions

1. Why is it important for public health professionals to develop foundational programming skills, even when GenAI tools like ChatGPT can generate code and assist with analysis?
2. How can ChatGPT be used effectively as a learning assistant in machine learning and R programming? What safeguards should be in place to ensure responsible use?
3. What are the key differences between supervised and unsupervised learning, and how might each be applied to solve different types of public health problems?
4. What role does explainability play in the responsible use of machine learning in public health? How can tools like R help improve model interpretability and stakeholder communication?
5. Imagine a case scenario where you are asked to apply machine learning to address substance use disorder (or another public health challenge) in your community. What type of data would you need? Which ML methods might be appropriate? How would you evaluate and communicate the results?

References

Alkaissi, H., & McFarlane, S. I. (2023). Artificial hallucinations in ChatGPT: Implications in scientific writing. *Cureus, 15*(2), e35179. https://doi.org/10.7759/cureus.35179

Bang, Y., Cahyawijaya, S., Lee, N., et al. (2023). A multitask, multilingual, multimodal evaluation of ChatGPT on reasoning, hallucination, and interactivity. *arXiv preprint*, arXiv:2302.04023. https://doi.org/10.48550/arXiv.2302.04023

Dwivedi, Y. K., et al. (2023). So what if ChatGPT wrote it? Multidisciplinary perspectives on opportunities, challenges, and implications of generative conversational AI for research, practice, and policy. *International Journal of Information Management, 71*, 102642. https://doi.org/10.1016/j.ijinfomgt.2023.102642

Hamilton, A. J., Strauss, A. T., Martinez, D. A., Hinson, J. S., Levin, S., Lin, G., & Klein, E. Y. (2021). Machine learning and artificial intelligence: Applications in healthcare epidemiology. *Antimicrobial Stewardship & Healthcare Epidemiology, 1*(1), e28. https://doi.org/10.1017/ash.2021.192

Kazemitabaar, M., Ye, R., Wang, X., Henley, A. Z., Denny, P., Craig, M., & Grossman, T. (2024). CodeAid: Evaluating a classroom deployment of an LLM-based programming assistant that balances student and educator needs. In *Proceedings of the 2024 CHI conference on human factors in computing systems (CHI '24)* (pp. 1–20). Association for Computing Machinery. https://doi.org/10.1145/3613904.3642773

Kung, T. H., Cheatham, M., Medenilla, A., Sillos, C., De Leon, L., et al. (2023). Performance of ChatGPT on USMLE: Potential for AI-assisted medical education using large language models. *PLOS Digital Health, 2*(2), e0000198. https://doi.org/10.1371/journal.pdig.0000198

Obermeyer, Z., & Emanuel, E. J. (2016). Predicting the future—Big data, machine learning, and clinical medicine. *New England Journal of Medicine, 375*(13), 1216–1219. https://doi.org/10.1056/NEJMp1606181

Peng, R. D. (2020). *R programming for data science*. Leanpub. https://leanpub.com/rprogramming

Sallam, M. (2023). ChatGPT utility in healthcare education, research, and practice: Systematic review on the promising perspectives and valid concerns. *Healthcare, 11*(6), 887. https://doi.org/10.3390/healthcare11060887

Topol, E. (2019). *Deep medicine: How artificial intelligence can make healthcare human again*. Basic Books.

Vaithilingam, P., Zhang, T., & Glassman, E. L. (2022). Expectation vs. experience: Evaluating the usability of code generation tools powered by large language models. In *Proceedings of the 2022 CHI conference on human factors in computing systems extended abstracts* (pp. 1–7). https://doi.org/10.1145/3491101.3519665

Chapter 2
Understanding AI and Machine Learning for Public Health

Learning Objectives
By the end of this chapter, readers will be able to:

1. **Define** core AI/ML terms like supervised and unsupervised learning.
2. **Describe** how AI/ML support public health tasks like surveillance, decision-making, and health promotion.
3. **Discuss** benefits and challenges of using electronic health records (EHRs) in AI-driven public health research.
4. **Evaluate** ethical and legal concerns in public health AI, including bias and regulation.
5. **Use** basic ML methods with EHR-like data in RStudio for applied health analysis.

Foundational Concepts

Building on the broad overview presented in Chap. 1, this chapter focuses on the foundational concepts of artificial intelligence (AI) and machine learning (ML) as they relate to public health practice. As introduced earlier, AI is transforming how we approach prevention, diagnosis, intervention, and system-level planning. Central to this transformation is the use of ML techniques that allow practitioners and researchers to analyze complex data, detect patterns, generate predictions, and support timely decision-making in diverse public health contexts (Rajkomar et al., 2019; Beam & Kohane, 2018).

The rise of ML in public health is closely linked to the explosive growth in the scale and diversity of health-related data—what many refer to as the "Big Data" era. Today's data sources extend well beyond traditional surveillance systems. They

---

Supplementary Information The online version contains supplementary material available at https://doi.org/10.1007/978-3-032-08677-8_2.

R. Leung, *Leveraging GenAI for Machine Learning Education in Public Health*,
https://doi.org/10.1007/978-3-032-08677-8_2

include electronic health records (EHRs), mobile health applications, wearable devices, environmental monitoring, social media platforms, and large-scale population surveys (Khoury et al., 2016). Together, these heterogeneous data streams offer unprecedented opportunities to track risk factors, monitor emerging health threats, evaluate interventions, and guide resource allocation with greater precision and timeliness (Chen et al., 2020).

Among these sources, EHRs stand out as a particularly rich and underutilized resource for ML applications in public health. Accelerated by the US HITECH Act of 2009, widespread adoption of EHR systems has led to the digitization of patient-level clinical data across health systems (Leung, 2012). EHRs contain extensive longitudinal data on demographics, diagnoses, treatments, outcomes, and service use—making them ideal for predictive modeling, population health surveillance, and health services research. Moreover, the integration of AI techniques such as natural language processing (NLP) allows for analysis of unstructured data (e.g., clinical notes and radiology reports), while computer vision enables the interpretation of medical images, and other ML tools support personalized care planning and delivery optimization (Vayena et al., 2018).

As public health evolves in a data-rich environment, the ability to derive actionable insights from complex, multimodal data is becoming essential. AI and ML provide the computational framework needed to harness these datasets in support of better health outcomes, reduced disparities, and more efficient systems (Obermeyer et al., 2019). At the same time, the deployment of these technologies must be accompanied by careful consideration of ethical issues such as data privacy, algorithmic fairness, and transparency—principles that are vital for fostering trust and ensuring responsible AI use (Char et al., 2020).

This chapter aims to equip readers with a solid foundation in AI and ML concepts relevant to public health. It introduces key terminology and model categories, explains the hierarchical relationships among AI, ML, and deep learning, and explores commonly used ML techniques. The chapter also introduces the concept of multimodal data integration and illustrates real-world public health use cases, using EHRs as a central example. Readers will be guided through practical coding exercises in RStudio using simulated data, with a focus on building not only technical proficiency but also ethical awareness and critical judgment essential for responsible application in the field.

Terminologies and Definitions

Having discussed the foundational role of AI and the growing importance of data-rich environments—particularly those involving electronic health records (EHRs)—it is now essential to clarify key terminologies that underpin this rapidly evolving field. This section introduces and distinguishes four core concepts frequently used in data science and public health analytics: *artificial intelligence (AI)*, *machine learning (ML)*, *deep learning (DL)*, and *large language models (LLMs)*. Understanding their definitions and hierarchical relationships provides a conceptual framework for engaging with the practical tools and methods introduced throughout the book.

Artificial intelligence (AI) is a broad field encompassing computational systems that perform tasks typically associated with human intelligence, such as reasoning, decision-making, pattern recognition, and natural language processing (Russell & Norvig, 2020). In public health, AI technologies are increasingly used to improve disease surveillance, streamline clinical workflows, and support real-time decision-making. For example, AI can analyze EHR data to identify patients at risk of hospital readmission or detect early warning signs of outbreaks across multiple data sources (Rajkomar et al., 2019).

Machine learning (ML) is a key subfield within AI focused on designing algorithms that learn from data and improve performance over time without being explicitly programmed (Murphy, 2012). Unlike traditional statistical models, which often rely on fixed assumptions, ML algorithms adaptively identify patterns in high-dimensional datasets. This flexibility makes ML particularly valuable for analyzing complex, heterogeneous sources such as EHRs. Applications in public health include predicting disease risk, optimizing resource allocation, and identifying health misinformation (Beam & Kohane, 2018; Chen et al., 2020).

Deep learning (DL) is a specialized branch of ML that uses multi-layered neural networks to detect intricate patterns in large-scale or unstructured data, such as images, speech, or free text. DL has been instrumental in recent advances in medical imaging, NLP, and multimodal data integration. In the context of EHRs, deep learning can be used to extract information from clinical notes, interpret radiological scans, and uncover complex associations across disparate data streams.

Large language models (LLMs)—such as ChatGPT—represent an advanced application of DL. Trained on extensive textual data, LLMs are capable of understanding and generating human-like language. Their public health applications include automating the analysis of clinical documentation, summarizing research literature, supporting patient communication, and, as discussed in Chap. 3, enhancing learning and programming through conversational interfaces.

Together, these technologies reflect a layered hierarchy: *AI* is the overarching concept; *ML* is a methodological subset; *DL* is a specialized class of ML; and *LLMs* are a powerful implementation of DL focused on language. These methods are particularly well-suited to today's multimodal data environment, where public health information flows from a wide range of sources—including EHRs, mobile apps, wearable devices, population surveys, and social media (Khoury et al., 2016; Obermeyer et al., 2019).

Understanding these terms—and how they relate to each other—is essential for navigating the ML methods and GenAI tools introduced in subsequent chapters. Figure 2.1 illustrates this hierarchical relationship, showing how each layer builds on the next to enable increasingly advanced capabilities for public health data analysis and decision-making.

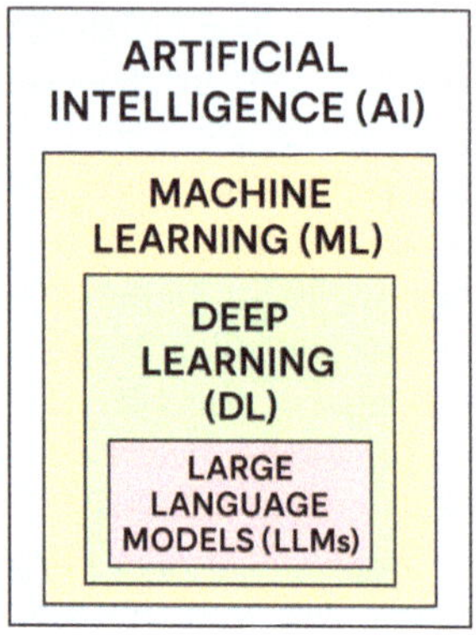

Fig. 2.1 Relationship between AI, ML, DL, and LLM

Key Types of Machine Learning Relevant to Public Health

Having introduced the core terminologies of *artificial intelligence (AI)*, *machine learning (ML)*, *deep learning (DL)*, and *large language models (LLMs)*—and clarified their hierarchical relationships—we now turn to the specific ML categories most relevant to public health practice. This section provides an accessible overview of foundational ML concepts, with a focus on practical, responsible application across diverse data environments.

Machine learning encompasses a wide array of modeling approaches. To navigate this landscape effectively, it is useful to distinguish four main categories: *supervised learning*, *unsupervised learning*, *semi-supervised learning*, and *reinforcement learning*. Understanding these categories allows practitioners to select appropriate models based on data structure, availability of labeled outcomes, and public health objectives.

Because this book is designed as an introductory resource, emphasis is placed on *supervised* and *unsupervised* learning—the two most commonly used and conceptually approachable forms of ML in public health. These methods are especially well-suited for working with rich datasets such as electronic health records (EHRs), health surveys, mobile health data, and environmental monitoring systems. The other two categories, *semi-supervised learning* and *reinforcement learning*, are introduced briefly to provide broader context, with more advanced discussions reserved for future study.

It is also important to recognize that each major category contains subtypes. For instance, supervised learning includes both *regression* models (used for continuous outcomes such as blood pressure or length of stay) and *classification* models (used for categorical outcomes such as disease presence or readmission risk). These distinctions will be explored further in subsequent chapters.

Supervised Learning—Supervised learning refers to training a model on a dataset that includes both input features and labeled outcomes. This category of ML is widely used in public health for predicting individual or population-level health risks, outcomes, or behaviors. For example, models can be trained to predict the onset of chronic diseases (e.g., diabetes or cardiovascular conditions) based on demographic, behavioral, and clinical data extracted from EHRs (Rajkomar et al., 2019).

Depending on the outcome type, supervised models may be framed as *regression* (predicting continuous values) or *classification* (predicting binary or multiclass labels). Practical use cases include classifying patients by hospitalization risk, estimating the number of emergency department visits, or predicting medication adherence. Supervised models have also been applied to mobile health data—such as GPS and accelerometer inputs—to anticipate behaviors like sedentariness or depressive episodes, thereby enabling early interventions (Fagherazzi et al., 2020).

Unsupervised Learning—Unsupervised learning involves analyzing data without pre-labeled outcomes. Instead, models detect natural patterns or structures within the dataset. This approach is valuable in exploratory public health research where subpopulations or hidden relationships need to be uncovered.

Clustering techniques are commonly used to group individuals by risk behavior profiles, geographic exposure, or social determinants of health, often using EHRs, administrative data, or population surveys. Dimensionality reduction techniques (e.g., principal component analysis) help simplify complex datasets while preserving essential structure, supporting visualization and subsequent modeling. Unsupervised learning is especially useful in contexts where labeling data is infeasible or the goal is pattern discovery rather than prediction (Chen et al., 2020).

Semi-supervised Learning—Semi-supervised learning combines a small amount of labeled data with a large pool of unlabeled data, leveraging both to build more robust models. This method is particularly useful when labeling data is costly or resource-intensive, as in genomic analysis, syndromic surveillance, or annotation of clinical notes in EHRs.

While promising for public health domains with limited labeled data, semi-supervised learning requires more technical expertise in model design and validation. For this reason, the concept is introduced briefly here, with more advanced treatment reserved for future volumes (Topol, 2019).

Reinforcement Learning—Reinforcement learning (RL) focuses on learning optimal actions through iterative interaction with a dynamic environment. The model receives feedback in the form of rewards or penalties and adapts its strategy to maximize long-term benefit.

In public health, RL has been used in emerging areas such as optimizing vaccine distribution logistics, designing adaptive behavioral interventions, and developing personalized management strategies for chronic diseases (Char et al., 2020). Despite its potential, RL involves complex modeling environments and evaluation methods, and is therefore introduced at a conceptual level in this book, with detailed applications left for more advanced study.

Figure 2.2 summarizes the key characteristics of each ML category. By understanding the distinctions between supervised, unsupervised, semi-supervised, and reinforcement learning—and their respective subtypes such as regression, classification, clustering, and dimensionality reduction—readers will be prepared to begin

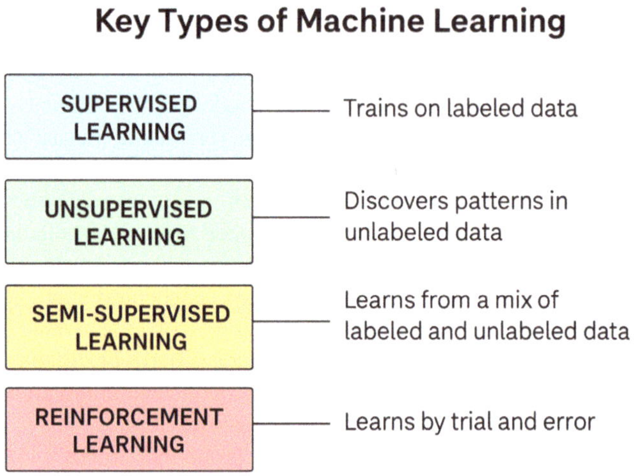

Fig. 2.2 Characteristics of ML models

applying ML methods to real-world public health problems using structured and unstructured data sources.

As an introductory resource, this book prioritizes hands-on guidance in *supervised learning* as a foundation for applied ML in public health. However, readers will also gain practical exposure to *unsupervised learning* techniques, introductory *natural language processing* (NLP) for clinical text analysis, and selected advanced models to broaden their analytical toolkit and inspire further exploration in healthcare data science.

ML for Public Health Enhancement: Electronic Health Records Studies

Electronic health records (EHRs) offer a rich and practical data source for exploring how machine learning (ML) can be applied in public health and clinical settings. EHRs contain a diverse range of structured and unstructured data routinely collected in healthcare environments, making them well-suited for the wide array of ML models introduced earlier in this chapter (Rajkomar et al., 2018).

EHR data typically include demographics such as age, sex, race, income, and insurance status, alongside comprehensive clinical records containing diagnoses, laboratory test results, vital signs, and medication histories. Additionally, EHRs capture behavioral indicators including substance use patterns, physical activity levels, and mental health screening results. Provider documentation—including care plans, discharge summaries, and free-text clinical notes—adds another layer of valuable information. Because EHRs reflect real-world, longitudinal patient trajectories, they serve as an ideal foundation for demonstrating how different ML techniques produce distinct types of insights (Choi et al., 2020).

Applications Across ML Types

The versatility of EHR data becomes apparent when considering how different ML approaches can extract various types of insights from the same dataset. Supervised learning can be used to predict outcomes such as hospital readmissions, risk of adverse drug events, or onset of chronic conditions based on historical patient characteristics. For example, a classification model might flag patients at high risk of 30-day readmission, while a regression model could estimate time until next appointment (Rajkomar et al., 2018; Shung et al., 2018).

Unsupervised learning helps uncover hidden subgroups within a patient population that may not be visible through traditional analysis. Clustering algorithms applied to EHRs might reveal distinct patterns in treatment response or identify unique chronic disease phenotypes, providing new insights into population health management (Choi et al., 2020; Beaulieu-Jones et al., 2019).

Semi-supervised learning becomes particularly relevant in EHR analysis when only a subset of patient records has labeled outcomes—for example, confirmed diagnosis codes—while a larger dataset remains unlabeled. This situation is common in population health surveillance, where manual chart review is resource-intensive but necessary for validation (Luo et al., 2022). Though more advanced, reinforcement learning may be applied to simulate and optimize clinical pathways, such as determining when to initiate a specific treatment plan for diabetes or when to escalate care intensity, supporting adaptive, decision-based modeling using EHR logs over time (Gottesman et al., 2019).

Potential Findings and Public Health Insights

When used responsibly, ML models trained on EHR data can support multiple aspects of public health practice and enhancement. Predictive analytics can anticipate disease progression, hospital utilization patterns, or gaps in preventive care, enabling proactive interventions that improve population health outcomes (Shung et al., 2018). These models can also provide clinical decision support by suggesting potential care recommendations or medication adjustments based on similar patient profiles, ultimately contributing to better health outcomes at both individual and community levels (Rajkomar et al., 2018). At the population level, EHR-based ML can stratify patients by risk, identify underserved groups, and optimize outreach efforts to improve health equity and address social determinants of health (Choi et al., 2020).

Key Challenges in EHR-Based ML Studies

Despite their utility, EHRs present several well-documented challenges that practitioners must navigate carefully when conducting ML studies. Data incompleteness and inconsistency are common issues, with missing lab results, outdated problem lists, and varying documentation practices creating gaps in the analytical foundation (Goldstein et al., 2016). Variability in data standards and coding practices across institutions further complicates model development and transferability, as models trained on one health system's data may not perform well when applied to another's (Rajkomar et al., 2018). Privacy and ethical concerns persist even with de-identified data, requiring robust governance frameworks and strict compliance with regulatory requirements, particularly when studies aim to inform public health policy (Murdoch & Detsky, 2013; Brisimi et al., 2024).

Pedagogical Approach: Using Simulated EHR Studies

To support experiential learning while maintaining ethical and regulatory standards, this book uses simulated EHR datasets that are modeled on real-world formats and complexities but contain no identifiable patient information (Yoon et al., 2023; Chen et al., 2023). This approach allows students to practice ML tasks using RStudio, work with realistic variable types and data structures, and develop reproducible workflows in a risk-free learning environment that mirrors actual public health research settings. The datasets can be downloaded here: https://livememphis-my.sharepoint.com/personal/rcleung_memphis_edu/_layouts/15/onedrive.aspx?id=%2Fpersonal%2Frcleung%5Fmemphis%5Fedu%2FDocuments%2FGenAI%20Book%20Datasets&ga=1

The use of synthetic EHR data addresses key privacy challenges while maintaining high fidelity to real clinical data patterns, enabling effective learning without compromising patient confidentiality (Yoon et al., 2023; Torfi & Fox, 2023). By using EHRs as a central case example throughout the book, learners will be able to connect ML techniques with practical, high-impact use cases that reflect current trends in healthcare and public health practice, preparing them to conduct meaningful studies that can enhance population health outcomes.

Expanding AI Modalities in Public Health: Beyond Traditional EHRs

In addition to machine learning applications with structured EHR data, AI encompasses a wider range of techniques that can be integrated with electronic health records to create more comprehensive health intelligence systems.

Multimodal AI Applications in Healthcare

Natural Language Processing (NLP) represents a powerful approach for extracting and analyzing health-related content from unstructured data sources such as provider notes, clinical documentation, and patient communications. When combined with EHR structured data, NLP can unlock insights from the vast amounts of free-text clinical notes, discharge summaries, and radiology reports that comprise up to 80% of health record content (Ford et al., 2016; Wang et al., 2024). This capability transforms previously inaccessible narrative information into actionable clinical intelligence.

Computer vision applications in healthcare include tasks such as skin cancer classification using images, fall detection in elder care settings, and analysis of radiological data for early disease diagnosis (Esteva et al., 2017; Liu et al., 2024). When integrated with EHR patient history and demographics, computer vision algorithms can provide more contextually-aware diagnostic support that considers both visual findings and clinical background.

Wearable and sensor integration offers continuous monitoring capabilities that provide real-time physiological data. These devices can be combined with longitudinal EHR records to create comprehensive patient profiles for chronic disease management and preventive care (Khanna et al., 2024; Peterson et al., 2024). This integration enables the transition from episodic care documentation to continuous health monitoring.

Predictive analytics leverages ML-powered models that combine EHR data with external data sources to forecast public health outcomes like hospital admissions, disease outbreaks, or resource utilization needs. These applications support real-time policymaking and resource allocation decisions by providing evidence-based projections (Shamout et al., 2021; Rahman et al., 2024).

Integration of Multiple Data Streams with EHRs

The increasing availability of biomedical data from large biobanks, electronic health records, medical imaging, wearable and ambient biosensors, and genomic sequencing has set the stage for multimodal AI solutions that capture the complexity of human health (Acosta et al., 2022). The promise of AI/ML lies in their ability to integrate heterogeneous health data from diverse sources with traditional EHR systems.

The core data integration framework positions clinical data from EHRs as the longitudinal backbone, providing structured diagnoses, medications, lab results, and care episodes. This foundation is enhanced through mobile and wearable data that offer continuous behavioral and physiological insights complementing episodic clinical encounters. Social determinants of health data, including housing, employment, and environmental factors, provide crucial context for understanding health outcomes. Additionally, genomic and biomarker data enable personalized medicine approaches when integrated with clinical phenotypes, while environmental data such as air quality and climate information supports tracking of ecological health risks and their correlation with clinical outcomes. Social media and digital health platforms contribute by monitoring population health trends, treatment adherence, and mental health indicators.

Enhanced EHR-Centric Applications

The Holistic AI in Medicine (HAIM) framework demonstrates how multimodal inputs can be systematically integrated with EHR data to enhance clinical decision-making (Moor et al., 2023). Key applications include comprehensive risk stratification that combines EHR clinical history with wearable device data and socioeconomic indicators to identify patients at risk for adverse outcomes with greater precision than clinical data alone.

Personalized treatment optimization represents another significant application, integrating pharmacogenomic data, treatment response patterns from EHRs, and real-time monitoring data to optimize medication selection and dosing for individual patients. Population health surveillance merges EHR disease surveillance with environmental monitoring, social media sentiment analysis, and mobility data for early outbreak detection and response planning.

Care coordination enhancement utilizes NLP to extract care plans from clinical notes, combined with patient-reported outcomes from mobile apps and wearable adherence monitoring, to support coordinated care delivery across multiple providers and settings.

Technical Implementation Considerations

The integration of multiple data streams with EHRs requires addressing several technical challenges. Data standardization ensures interoperability between diverse data formats, coding systems, and temporal resolutions, enabling seamless integration across platforms. Privacy-preserving integration implements federated learning and differential privacy techniques to enable multi-source analysis while protecting individual privacy and maintaining regulatory compliance.

Real-time processing capabilities require developing architectures capable of processing streaming data from wearables and sensors alongside static EHR records, ensuring timely insights for clinical decision-making. Bias mitigation addresses potential algorithmic bias when combining data sources with different representation patterns and collection methodologies, promoting equitable outcomes across diverse populations.

When designed ethically and implemented responsibly, these integrated systems can support evidence-based and scalable public health interventions that leverage the full spectrum of available health information (Obermeyer et al., 2019; Rajpurkar et al., 2024).

Core Challenges in EHR-Based AI Implementation

Data Quality, Bias, and Interoperability

The integration of AI and machine learning into public health practices—especially those involving electronic health records (EHRs)—brings substantial promise, but it also introduces a set of persistent data-related challenges. EHRs often contain incomplete, inconsistent, or outdated information, such as missing lab results or unverified problem lists, which can compromise the performance of predictive models. Additionally, data fragmentation across health systems, coupled with a lack of interoperability and standardized formats, hinders the development of generalizable algorithms and limits population-level insights. Models trained in specific institutional contexts (e.g., urban academic centers) may not perform reliably in rural or under-resourced environments. These challenges also intersect with concerns about algorithmic fairness: models trained on biased or incomplete datasets can inadvertently reinforce health disparities, particularly for underrepresented populations (Obermeyer et al., 2019). Without rigorous auditing and quality assurance, AI risks deepening existing inequities rather than addressing them.

Workforce Development as a Foundational Challenge

Beyond technical hurdles, workforce readiness remains one of the most important but underappreciated conditions for successful AI implementation in public health. As machine learning applications become more accessible, there is a growing need to equip the public health workforce with practical data skills, including the ability to interpret and apply AI-generated outputs. This book responds directly to that need. By focusing on machine learning programming in R, it aims to empower public health professionals with the competencies required to engage with AI tools meaningfully and responsibly. Workforce development is not just an implementation barrier—it is central to unlocking the full utility of ML and EHR integration.

Ethical and Responsible Use of AI and GenAI

Equally critical is the need for public health professionals to understand the limitations of both traditional ML methods and emerging GenAI tools. While GenAI platforms such as ChatGPT, Claude, and Copilot can simplify programming tasks and support learning, they also present new risks. These systems may hallucinate information, obscure decision logic, or reinforce biases in subtle ways. Effective public health practice requires more than technical capability—it demands critical reflection on how, when, and why these technologies are used. Ethical concerns related to privacy, transparency, and accountability must be addressed through careful system design, regulatory compliance, and institutional governance (Dwivedi et al., 2024). Furthermore, black-box models may not be appropriate for policy settings where interpretability and evidence-based decision-making are essential.

Organizational Capacity and Infrastructure

To support the responsible use of AI, organizations must invest in robust infrastructure. This includes technical systems that support real-time data integration from multiple sources (e.g., EHRs, wearables, environmental sensors), as well as governance frameworks that ensure data quality, traceability, and privacy. At the leadership level, health entities must develop cohesive AI strategies that balance innovation with safety and regulatory requirements. These systems should be built not only for current needs but with scalability in mind, capable of adapting to future data sources and analytic methods.

Reflections and Future Possibilities

The application of AI and ML in public health is no longer theoretical—it is actively reshaping how we understand, monitor, and improve population health. This chapter began by clarifying the often-misunderstood concepts of artificial intelligence and machine learning, distinguishing between supervised, unsupervised, semi-supervised, and reinforcement learning as practical tools for addressing diverse public health problems. We focused particularly on the value and limitations of electronic health record (EHR) data, showing how ML methods can uncover patterns in clinical, behavioral, and demographic indicators, and how these insights can guide timely and equitable interventions.

Beyond EHRs, we explored the expanding frontier of multimodal data integration. Public health is increasingly benefiting from the convergence of data streams—natural language processing of provider notes, wearable sensor data, computer vision for diagnostic imaging, and environmental exposure data—all of which can be linked with EHRs to create richer, more contextualized models of health and disease. The HAIM framework and other architectures illustrate how public health intelligence is being enhanced by combining modalities once siloed from one another.

However, we also emphasized that successful implementation depends on more than just data and algorithms. It requires strong institutional infrastructure, cross-disciplinary collaboration, and most critically, workforce development. One of the major themes of this chapter is that the potential of AI in public health will remain underutilized unless professionals are equipped not only with technical skills but also with the judgment and ethical awareness to apply them responsibly. This includes understanding data bias, ensuring algorithmic fairness, navigating privacy concerns, and developing scalable implementation strategies that prioritize community engagement.

The simulated EHR datasets provided in this book serve as a foundational tool for hands-on learning, allowing readers to build confidence in programming with R and applying core ML techniques. These exercises are designed not only to reinforce conceptual understanding but to provide a safe, ethical environment to engage with real-world data challenges.

As we look ahead, the role of AI in public health is expected to deepen and diversify. Future applications may include computer vision to improve early cancer diagnosis, synthetic data simulations to enhance medical education and drug discovery, and predictive models to support preventive health, mental wellness, and chronic disease management. Additional use cases are emerging in domains such as substance use disorder prevention and treatment, mental health and stress monitoring through passive data collection, maternal and child health risk prediction, and dietary assessment using AI-enabled image recognition of food. Even agricultural and food system innovations—such as optimizing crop yields, tracking nutrition quality, and improving food access—are increasingly benefiting from AI-driven analytics.

AI techniques are also being explored in addressing broader societal issues—such as reducing gun violence, assessing climate change risks, promoting sustainability, and enhancing cybersecurity in health infrastructure.

Ultimately, the future of public health will be shaped by how well we integrate emerging technologies with a grounded understanding of public needs, ethical standards, and system constraints. As we move forward, this book aims to prepare readers to participate actively in that future—bringing technical rigor, ethical clarity, and a deep commitment to equity into every application of AI and machine learning in public health.

Discussion Questions

1. What are the key differences between supervised and unsupervised machine learning, and how can each be applied in a public health context?
2. In what ways can algorithmic bias affect the outcomes of public health interventions? Provide examples.

3. What are some of the privacy concerns when using real EHR data in public health research? How can simulated data help address these concerns?
4. How can interdisciplinary collaboration improve the development and implementation of AI tools in public health?
5. What are the essential elements of an ethical AI framework for public health?

References

Acosta, J. N., Falcone, G. J., Rajpurkar, P., & Topol, E. J. (2022). Multimodal biomedical AI. *Nature Medicine, 28*(9), 1773–1784. https://www.nature.com/articles/s41591-022-01981-2

Beam, A. L., & Kohane, I. S. (2018). Big data and machine learning in health care. *JAMA, 319*(13), 1317–1318. https://doi.org/10.1001/jama.2017.18391

Beaulieu-Jones, B. K., Finlayson, S. G., Yuan, W., Altman, R. B., Kohane, I. S., Prasad, V., & Yu, K. H. (2019). Examining the use of real-world evidence in the regulatory process. *Clinical Pharmacology & Therapeutics, 107*(4), 843–852. https://www.nature.com/articles/s41746-020-0301-z

Brisimi, T. S., Xu, T., Wang, T., Dai, W., & Chen, W. (2024). Balancing privacy and progress: A review of privacy challenges, systemic oversight, and patient perceptions in AI-driven healthcare. *Applied Sciences, 14*(2), 675. https://www.mdpi.com/2076-3417/14/2/675

Char, D. S., Abràmoff, M. D., & Shah, N. H. (2020). Implementing machine learning in health care — Addressing ethical challenges. *New England Journal of Medicine, 378*(11), 981–983. https://doi.org/10.1056/NEJMp1714229

Chen, E., Lerman, K., & Ferrara, E. (2020). Tracking social media discourse about the COVID-19 pandemic: Development of a public coronavirus Twitter data set. *JMIR Public Health and Surveillance, 6*(2), e19273. https://publichealth.jmir.org/2020/2/e19273

Chen, R. J., Lu, M. Y., Wang, J., Williamson, D. F., Rodig, S. J., Lindeman, N. I., & Mahmood, F. (2023). Synthetic data in health care: A narrative review. *PLOS Digital Health, 2*(1), e0000082. https://www.ncbi.nlm.nih.gov/pmc/articles/PMC9931305/

Chen, S., Zhou, Z., Yang, S., & Xing, L. (2020). Digital health for aging populations. *Nature Medicine, 26*(11), 1623–1630. https://www.nature.com/articles/s41591-020-1088-9

Choi, E., Bahadori, M. T., Schuetz, A., Stewart, W. F., & Sun, J. (2020). Deep representation learning of electronic health records to unlock patient stratification at scale. *npj Digital Medicine, 3*(1), 96. https://www.nature.com/articles/s41746-020-0301-z

Dwivedi, D. N., Mahanty, G., & Dwivedi, V. N. (2024). Ethical AI Assessment: A Framework with Composite Scores. In International Conference on Computing and Machine Learning (pp. 497–511). Singapore: Springer Nature Singapore. https://link.springer.com/chapter/10.1007/978-981-97-6588-1_37

Esteva, A., Kuprel, B., Novoa, R. A., Ko, J., Swetter, S. M., Blau, H. M., & Thrun, S. (2017). Dermatologist-level classification of skin cancer with deep neural networks. *Nature, 542*(7639), 115–118. https://www.nature.com/articles/nature21056

Fagherazzi, G., Goetzinger, C., Rashid, M. A., Aguayo, G. A., & Huiart, L. (2020). Digital health strategies to fight COVID-19 worldwide: Challenges, recommendations, and a call for papers. *Journal of Medical Internet Research, 22*(6), e19284. https://doi.org/10.2196/19284

Ford, E., Carroll, J. A., Smith, H. E., Scott, D., & Cassell, J. A. (2016). Extracting information from the text of electronic medical records to improve case detection: A systematic review. *Journal of the American Medical Informatics Association, 23*(5), 1007–1015. https://pubmed.ncbi.nlm.nih.gov/27026615/

Goldstein, B. A., Navar, A. M., Pencina, M. J., & Ioannidis, J. P. (2016). Opportunities and challenges in developing risk prediction models with electronic health records data: A systematic review. *Journal of the American Medical Informatics Association, 24*(1), 198–208. https://pubmed.ncbi.nlm.nih.gov/37783537/

Gottesman, O., Johansson, F., Komorowski, M., Faisal, A., Sontag, D., Doshi-Velez, F., & Celi, L. A. (2019). Guidelines for reinforcement learning in healthcare. *Nature Medicine, 25*(1), 16–18. https://www.nature.com/articles/s41746-018-0029-1

Khanna, S., Sattar, A., & Hansen, D. (2024). A comprehensive review on advancements in wearable technologies: Revolutionizing cardiovascular medicine. *Cureus, 16*(6), e62384. https://pmc.ncbi.nlm.nih.gov/articles/PMC11212841/

Khoury, M. J., Iademarco, M. F., & Riley, W. T. (2016). Precision public health for the era of precision medicine. *American Journal of Preventive Medicine, 50*(3), 398–401. https://www.ajpmonline.org/article/S0749-3797(15)00506-X/fulltext

Leung, R. C. (2012). Health information technology and dynamic capabilities. *Health Care Management Review, 37*(1), 43–53. https://journals.lww.com/hcmrjournal/abstract/2012/01000/health_information_technology_and_dynamic.6.aspx

Liu, Y., Chen, A., Shi, L., Wang, J., & Li, X. (2024). Computer vision to enhance healthcare domain: An overview of features, implementation, and opportunities. *Digital Health, 10*, 20552076241256849. https://www.sciencedirect.com/science/article/pii/S2949866X24000662

Luo, Y., Peng, J., & Ma, S. (2022). Machine learning approaches for electronic health records phenotyping: A methodical review. *medRxiv*. https://www.medrxiv.org/content/10.1101/2022.04.23.22274218v1.full

Moor, M., Huang, B., Rieck, B., Horn, M., Rieck, T., Borgwardt, K., et al. (2023). Integrated multimodal artificial intelligence framework for healthcare applications. *npj Digital Medicine, 6*(1), 129. https://www.nature.com/articles/s41746-022-00689-4

Murdoch, T. B., & Detsky, A. S. (2013). The inevitable application of big data to health care. *JAMA, 309*(13), 1351–1352. https://www.ncbi.nlm.nih.gov/books/NBK551878/

Murphy, K. P. (2012). *Machine learning: A probabilistic perspective*. MIT Press. https://probml.github.io/pml-book/book1.html

Obermeyer, Z., Powers, B., Vogeli, C., & Mullainathan, S. (2019). Dissecting racial bias in an algorithm used to manage the health of populations. *Science, 366*(6464), 447–453. https://www.science.org/doi/10.1126/science.aax2342

Peterson, K., Martinez, R., & Thompson, D. (2024). The latest trends in wearable technology for healthcare. *HealthTech Magazine*. https://healthtechmagazine.net/article/2024/03/trends-wearable-technology-for-healthcare-perfcon

Rahman, M. S., Islam, M. R., Alam, M. S., Islam, I., Hoque, M. N., Akter, S., et al. (2024). Machine learning driven analysis of large scale multiomics data reveals functionally important genes for COVID-19 severity. *Scientific Reports, 14*(1), 5379. https://www.nature.com/articles/s41598-024-55439-1

Rajkomar, A., Dean, J., & Kohane, I. (2019). Machine learning in medicine. *New England Journal of Medicine, 380*(14), 1347–1358. https://www.nejm.org/doi/full/10.1056/NEJMra1814259

Rajkomar, A., Oren, E., Chen, K., Dai, A. M., Hajaj, N., Hardt, M., et al. (2018). Scalable and accurate deep learning with electronic health records. *npj Digital Medicine, 1*(1), 18. https://www.nature.com/articles/s41746-018-0029-1

Rajpurkar, P., Chen, E., Banerjee, O., & Topol, E. J. (2024). The future of healthcare using multimodal AI: Technology that can read, see, hear and sense. *Computer Methods and Programs in Biomedicine Update, 4*, 100146. https://www.sciencedirect.com/science/article/pii/S2772906024001869

Russell, S., & Norvig, P. (2020). *Artificial intelligence: A modern approach* (4th ed.). Pearson. https://aima.cs.berkeley.edu

Shamout, F. E., Shen, Y., Wu, N., Kaku, A., Park, J., Nakamura, T., et al. (2021). An artificial intelligence system for predicting the deterioration of COVID-19 patients in the emergency department. *npj Digital Medicine, 4*(1), 80. https://www.nature.com/articles/s41746-021-00453-0

Shung, D., Simonov, M., Gentry, M., Au, B., & Laine, L. (2018). Machine learning models in electronic health records can outperform conventional survival models for predicting patient mortality in coronary artery disease. *European Heart Journal, 40*(48), 3997–4006. https://www.ncbi.nlm.nih.gov/pmc/articles/PMC6118376/

Topol, E. (2019). *Deep medicine: How artificial intelligence can make healthcare human again*. Basic Books. https://www.basicbooks.com/titles/eric-topol/deep-medicine/9781541644649/

Torfi, A., & Fox, E. A. (2023). Harnessing the power of synthetic data in healthcare: Innovation, application, and privacy. *npj Digital Medicine, 6*(1), 186. https://www.nature.com/articles/s41746-023-00927-3

Vayena, E., Blasimme, A., & Cohen, I. G. (2018). Machine learning in medicine: Addressing ethical challenges. *PLoS Medicine, 15*(11), e1002689. https://doi.org/10.1371/journal.pmed.1002689

Wang, L., Zhang, Y., Wang, D., Tong, X., Liu, T., Zhang, S., et al. (2024). NLP in healthcare: Transforming patient care and efficiency. *Journal of Medical Internet Research, 26*(8), e45123. https://appinventiv.com/blog/nlp-in-healthcare/

Yoon, J., Drumright, L. N., & van der Schaar, M. (2023). EHR-safe: Generating high-fidelity and privacy-preserving synthetic electronic health records. *npj Digital Medicine, 6*(1), 141. https://www.nature.com/articles/s41746-023-00888-7

Chapter 3
Getting Started with ChatGPT and RStudio

Learning Objectives
By the end of this chapter, readers will be able to:

1. **Distinguish** between R and RStudio and their roles in public health data analysis.
2. **Install** and configure R/RStudio for data analysis and machine learning tasks.
3. **Write** basic R code to perform operations, assign variables, and create vectors.
4. **Load** built-in and external datasets using R functions.
5. **Use** ChatGPT to support R programming, code generation, and troubleshooting.

Introduction

Machine learning (ML) in public health relies on powerful statistical software to analyze complex datasets and develop predictive models. Commonly used tools include Python, R, and Excel—each with unique advantages (Cunningham et al., 2021). This book focuses on R because it is open-source, widely supported, and offers a rich ecosystem of packages ideal for statistical modeling, visualization, and integration with public health data. While Python and Excel may be covered in future resources, this book provides a foundation for learning ML in public health using R.

R is a widely used open-source programming language for statistical computing, data analysis, and visualization. Its relevance in public health spans epidemiological modeling, biostatistics, and machine learning (R Core Team, 2023). However, the command-line interface of R can be intimidating for beginners.

RStudio, an integrated development environment (IDE), addresses this challenge by offering a user-friendly interface. It features tools for visualization, debugging,

Supplementary Information The online version contains supplementary material available at https://doi.org/10.1007/978-3-032-08677-8_3.

R. Leung, *Leveraging GenAI for Machine Learning Education in Public Health*,
https://doi.org/10.1007/978-3-032-08677-8_3

and package management, which simplify the R programming process. For public health professionals new to programming, RStudio significantly enhances workflow efficiency and makes data analysis more approachable (RStudio, PBC, 2023).

This book also introduces the use of ChatGPT as an instructional companion. Throughout the chapters, ChatGPT is deliberately prompted to demonstrate coding techniques, explain RStudio features, clarify ML concepts, and assist with public health data analysis. In this way, ChatGPT serves as a conversational assistant, helping readers develop practical R programming skills and understand the applications of machine learning in public health.

Key Differences Between R and RStudio

R is the core programming language and computational environment. It provides essential statistical and graphical functions for data analysis. R can be used independently through a command-line interface or within text editors.

RStudio is an IDE that enhances working with R. It offers features like syntax highlighting, built-in package management, and an integrated help system. Unlike R, RStudio does not perform computations itself—it serves as a convenient interface for writing and executing R code.

Public health professionals use R and RStudio for tasks such as disease surveillance, predictive modeling, and health policy evaluation. While R provides strong computational capabilities, RStudio improves accessibility and workflow efficiency. Together, they are essential tools for researchers, helping to analyze large datasets and apply ML in epidemiology and biostatistics (R Core Team, 2023; RStudio, PBC, 2023). Table 3.1 summarizes the differences between the two:

Installing R and RStudio

To get started, users must first install R, available from the Comprehensive R Archive Network (CRAN) at https://cran.r-project.org. Choose the version appropriate for your operating system (Windows, macOS, or Linux). As of this writing, the latest version for Mac was 4.4.2 (2024-10-31). To begin, the following section provides a standard, step-by-step installation guide without using ChatGPT. In the next section, we will show how ChatGPT can generate the same instructions interactively based on a simple prompt.

Once R is installed (Fig. 3.1), the next step is to install RStudio, which provides an intuitive graphical interface for working with R. RStudio can be downloaded from the official RStudio website at https://posit.co/download/rstudio-desktop/. Users should select the free desktop version unless they require professional features. After downloading, follow the installation prompts to complete the setup. As of this publication, the latest version of RStudio for Mac was 2024.12.1 Build 563.

Table 3.1 Comparison between R and RStudio

Feature	R	RStudio
Definition	A programming language and environment for statistical computing.	An integrated development environment (IDE) designed to work with R.
Function	Performs data analysis, modeling, and visualization.	Provides tools for writing, organizing, and running R code efficiently.
User Interface	Command-line interface (text-based).	Graphical interface with panels for scripts, console, plots, etc.
Usability	More challenging for beginners due to lack of visual structure.	User-friendly and designed to simplify coding tasks and navigation.
Computation	Executes statistical functions and ML algorithms.	Does not compute; it sends instructions to R for execution.
Package management	Uses `install.packages()` and `library()` in the console.	Offers a graphical interface to manage packages more easily.
Visualization	Supports plotting through code.	Includes built-in plotting pane for previewing graphics.
Documentation access	Helps system accessible via? `function_name`.	Integrated help tab and searchable documentation pane.
File management	Code and data handled through file paths and console.	Project-based interface that organizes scripts, data, and outputs.
Where to download	https://cran.r-project.org	https://posit.co/download/rstudio-desktop/
Best use case	Core engine for executing statistical tasks.	Ideal interface for developing, testing, and managing R-based projects.

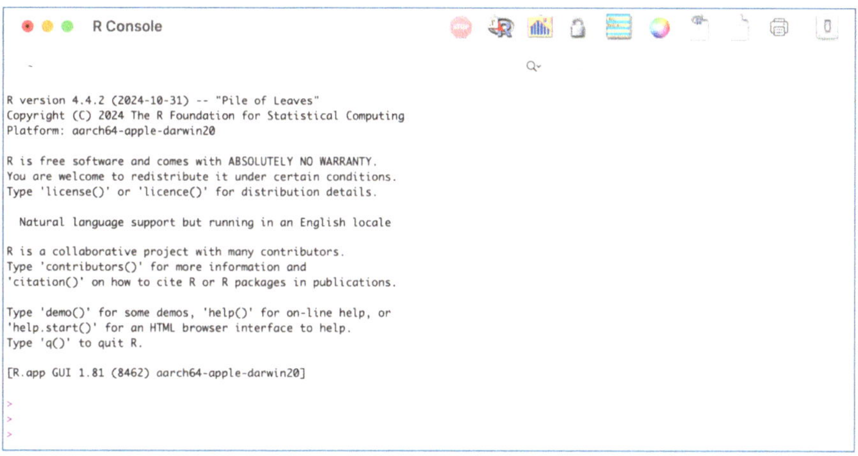

Fig. 3.1 The R interface

After installation, open RStudio. On a Mac, users can drag the RStudio icon to the dock for easy access. Upon launching RStudio, users will see an interface similar to Fig. 3.2. The environment consists of multiple panels: the **console** (lower left), **environment/history** (upper right), and **plots/viewer** (lower right). The **script**

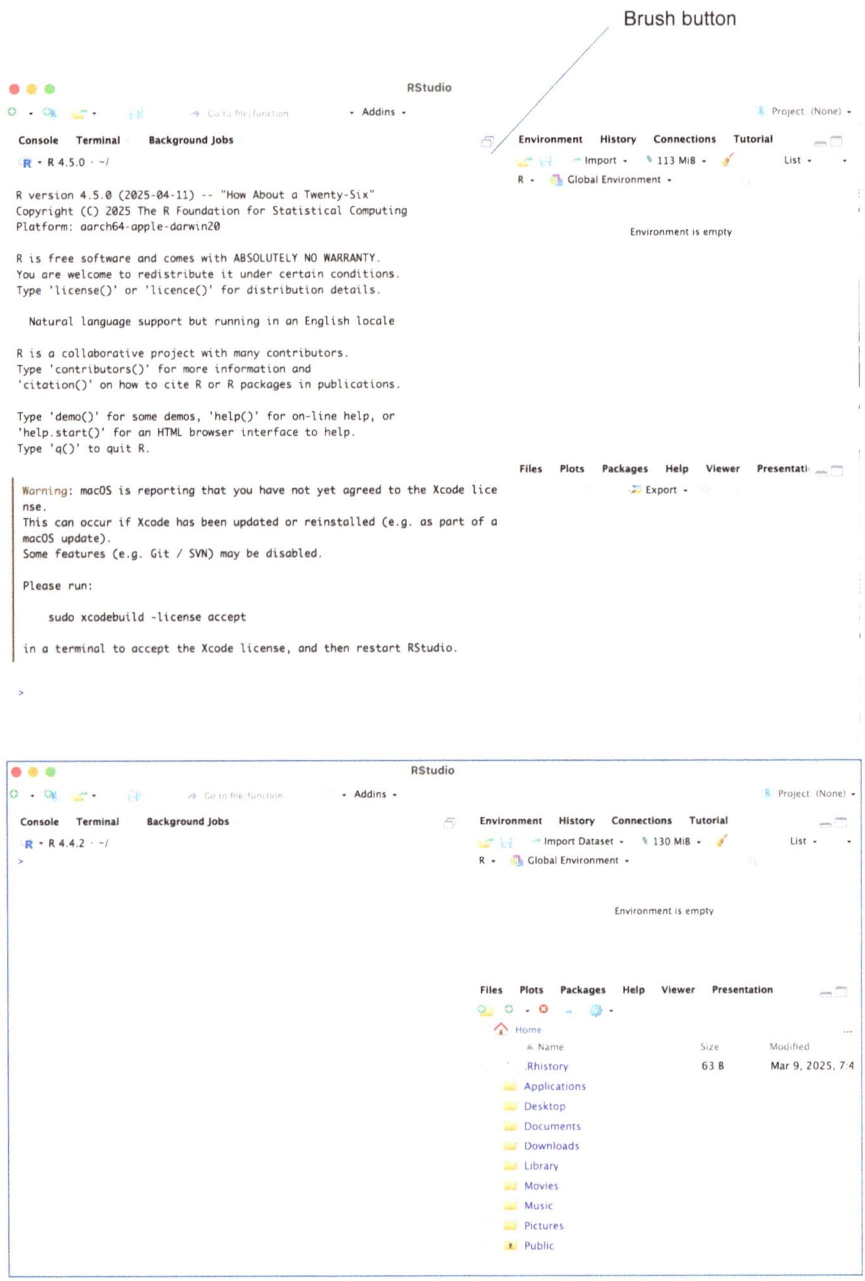

Fig. 3.2 The RStudio interface

editor will appear only after the user enters or opens a script. Each panel includes functional tools that enhance usability. For example, the brush icon in the upper-right corner of the console or environment panel allows users to clear content, helping maintain an organized workspace. After clicking this brush icon, the display will be refreshed—as illustrated when comparing the upper and lower views of Fig. 3.2.

Other tools—such as buttons for running scripts, managing packages, and saving outputs—contribute to an efficient and streamlined workflow. Together, these panels and features support effective data analysis and machine learning development in RStudio.

Installing and Loading Packages

To apply ML in R or RStudio, you'll need to install essential packages. For example, the caret package supports ML model training, and ggplot2 enables advanced data visualization. Installing these packages can be accomplished using the install.packages() function in R or RStudio (see Fig. 3.3):

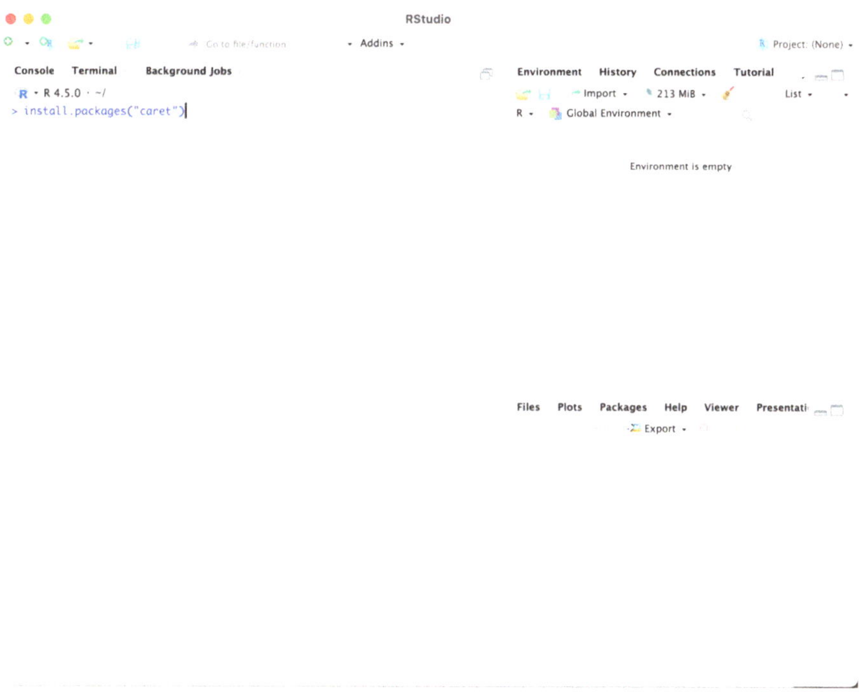

Fig. 3.3 Installation of the caret and ggplot2 packages

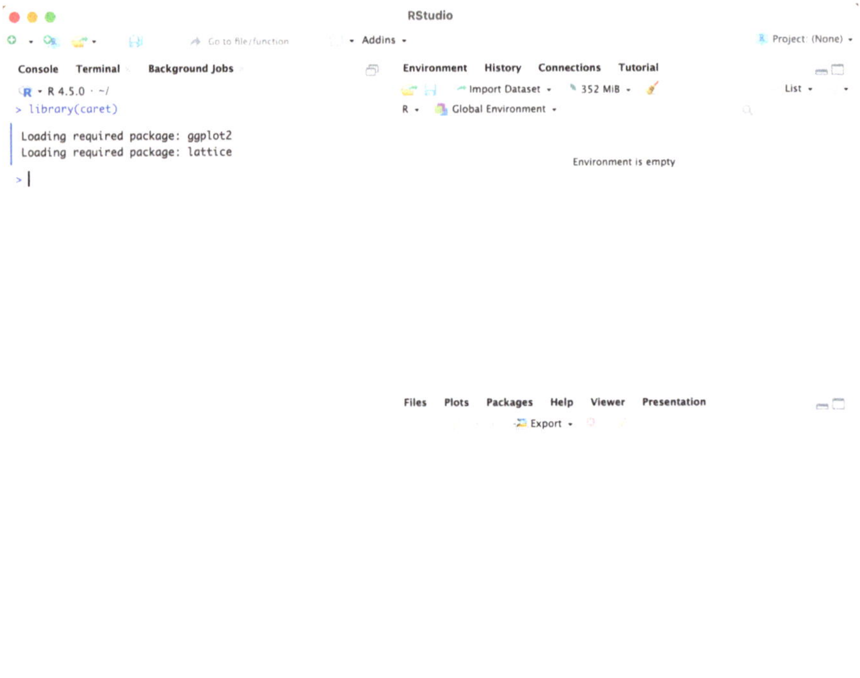

Fig. 3.4 The library function to load the installed packages

Once installed, these packages must be loaded using the library() function to ensure they are accessible during an analysis session. That is, type library(caret), as shown in Fig. 3.4:

Packages such as caret and ggplot2 will enable users to handle public health data efficiently and apply ML techniques for modeling and visualization.

Writing and Running Scripts

The script window in RStudio, mentioned earlier in this section, is where users can write, edit, and save R code for repeated use. This window supports structured coding, making it easier to organize, test, and manage multiple lines of code. Key buttons include **Save**, which allows you to store your script as an `.R` file, and **Run**, which executes the selected line or block of code directly in the console. Scripts created in this window can be edited and reused across different projects, supporting efficiency and reproducibility in data analysis. Figure 3.5 illustrates this feature using a sample script on basic arithmetic operations, which will be discussed in greater detail in later sections.

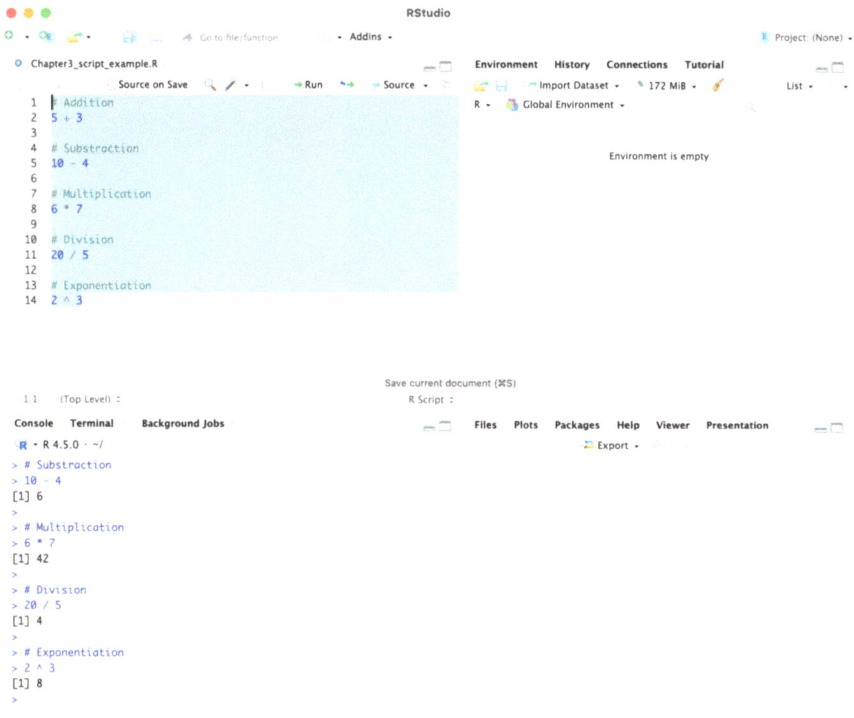

Fig. 3.5 The script window in RStudio

Role of ChatGPT

Figures in this chapter provide a visual walkthrough of R and RStudio. Now let's see how ChatGPT can support learning. If you visit ChatGPT (https://chatgpt.com/), you will see an interface like an open window. In this figure, you can see a box labeled "Ask anything" under the header "What can I help with?". This is the space where you can enter your prompt.

If you don't know how to install R or RStudio, you can type the prompt: "Provide step-by-step instructions to install R and RStudio on my computer, including how to verify the installation." ChatGPT will return clear, detailed steps. Prompts like this also work for coding, debugging, and understanding ML concepts.

ChatGPT will return the results as shown in Fig. 3.6.

The previous section provides a quick illustration of how we can use ChatGPT to learn about new software—namely, R and RStudio—from installation to simple coding commands. Additionally, you can ask for troubleshooting tips if you encounter any issues during the process. To use ChatGPT effectively, it is important to provide a clear prompt. For example, instead of asking "How do I install R and RStudio?", you can enter a more specific prompt in ChatGPT such as "Provide step-by-step instructions to install R and RStudio on my computer, including how to

Here is a step-by-step guide to install **R** and **RStudio** on your computer. These instructions apply to Windows, macOS, and Linux.

Step 1: Install R

R is the programming language. RStudio requires R to run.

For Windows:

1. Go to: https://cran.r-project.org
2. Click on **"Download R for Windows"**.
3. Click on **"base"**, then click **"Download R [version number] for Windows"**.
4. Open the downloaded `.exe` file and follow the installation prompts (default options are usually fine).

For macOS:

1. Go to: https://cran.r-project.org
2. Click on **"Download R for macOS"**.
3. Download the `.pkg` file for the latest R release (make sure it matches your macOS version).
4. Double-click the `.pkg` file and follow the installation prompts.

For Linux (Ubuntu/Debian):

Open a terminal and run the following commands:

bash Copy Edit

```bash
sudo apt update
sudo apt install r-base
```

Fig. 3.6 Results generated by ChatGPT regarding RStudio installation

verify the installation." Prompting has become a very important skill as the use of generative AI has increased its prevalence in society (OpenAI, n.d.). Below we will show a few examples. Additionally, we will discuss the importance of proper prompting in greater detail for generating ML codes in later chapters of this book. For the previous example regarding R and RStudio, the use of a very specific prompt does not make a big difference.

Step 2: Install RStudio

RStudio is an integrated development environment (IDE) that makes using R easier.

1. Go to: https://posit.co/download/rstudio-desktop/
2. Scroll down to **"RStudio Desktop (Open Source)"** and click **"Download"**.
3. Select your operating system (Windows, macOS, or Linux) and download the installer.
4. Open the downloaded file and follow the installation prompts.

Step 3: Launch RStudio

After installation:

- Open **RStudio** (not the R console).
- RStudio will detect your installed R version automatically.
- You're now ready to start coding in R.

Optional: Install Common Packages

After opening RStudio, run the following in the Console to install useful packages:

r Copy Edit

```r
install.packages(c("tidyverse", "data.table", "ggplot2", "readr"))
```

Let me know if you'd like help setting up specific R packages or running your first script.

Fig. 3.6 (continued)

Demonstrate R Syntax by Prompting

To demonstrate how ChatGPT assists in learning R syntax, we can jump right into using it to provide simple coding examples. Let's try the following prompt:

Provide simple R studio coding examples

The prompt returns a list of examples. Figure 3.7 provides the first three examples:

The codes shown in Fig. 3.7 work for both R and RStudio. Assume that we use RStudio. The first set of codes above shows how codes are entered in RStudio to perform basic arithmetic operations. The "#" sign is to indicate a comment line. For example, "# Addition" indicates that this line is only a comment. RStudio does not

Here are some simple R coding examples for RStudio:

1. Basic Arithmetic Operations

r Copy Edit

```r
# Addition
5 + 3

# Subtraction
10 - 4

# Multiplication
6 * 7

# Division
20 / 5

# Exponentiation
2^3
```

2. Assigning Variables

r Copy Edit

```r
x <- 10
y <- 5
z <- x + y
print(z)
```

3. Creating a Vector

r Copy Edit

```r
numbers <- c(1, 2, 3, 4, 5)
print(numbers)
```

Fig. 3.7 Simple R/RStudio codes generated by ChatGPT

perform any function for this line. Entering the second line, “5 + 3,” will return 8 in RStudio.

The second set is about assigning variables, using the <− assignment operator. For example, the line “x <- 10” means that the variable x is assigned the value 10, and the line “y <- 5” means that the variable y is assigned the value 5. The third set is about creating vectors. In the example above, the vector “numbers” is assigned a list of values that contain 1, 2, 3, 4, and 5. Users can use the Copy button at the upper-right corner of each set to copy the codes, paste them in RStudio, and run them. Doing so should give novice users a sense of how RStudio works. We will use more complex examples in later chapters.

Where Do We Get Data?

Public health professionals typically work with datasets that are more complex than the numbers shown in Fig. 3.7. For educational and demonstration purposes, RStudio provides a variety of built-in datasets, available either within the base software or through specific packages. Some of these built-in datasets will be useful for illustrating machine learning (ML) algorithms in this book. As mentioned, this book will also utilize a simulated electronic health records (EHR) dataset containing 500 observations and 10 variables, including patient demographics, clinical measurements, and health risk factors.

Built-in Data

Among the various built-in datasets available in base R and RStudio, the iris dataset is widely used to illustrate machine learning (ML) algorithms [Add reference]. The dataset has been extensively referenced to demonstrate classification problems, particularly such as decision trees and support vector machines (Fisher, 1936). In Chap. 4, we will use the iris dataset to demonstrate the K-Nearest Neighbors (KNN) algorithm and other ML techniques.

Some datasets are built into specific R packages, requiring users to first install the package and then load it using the library() function before accessing the data. The following section provides an example of how to work with such datasets in RStudio. In ChatGPT, use the prompt:

If we are interested in specific datasets such as "iris" and "BreastCancer" (within the mlbench package), we can prompt "Explain how RStudio uses built-in data" in ChatGPT. Figure 3.8 illustrates the results:

It is also possible to learn how R/RStudio loads built-in data such as "iris" and "breastcancer." Using the prompt of "provide coding in R for loading iris and BreastCancer datasets" will produce the results generated in Fig. 3.9:

In RStudio, datasets can be loaded using the data() function. For example, the iris dataset can be loaded with data(iris), and its first few rows can be displayed using head(iris). For the BreastCancer dataset, users must first install the mlbench package and load it into RStudio. Once the package is loaded, the dataset can be accessed using data(BreastCancer) (in some versions of RStudio, the quotation marks are necessary. So, type data("BreastCancer"). RStudio recognizes iris as a built-in dataset and BreastCancer as a dataset available within the mlbench package. However, users cannot reference a dataset using data() unless it is either built into R or explicitly loaded from a package.

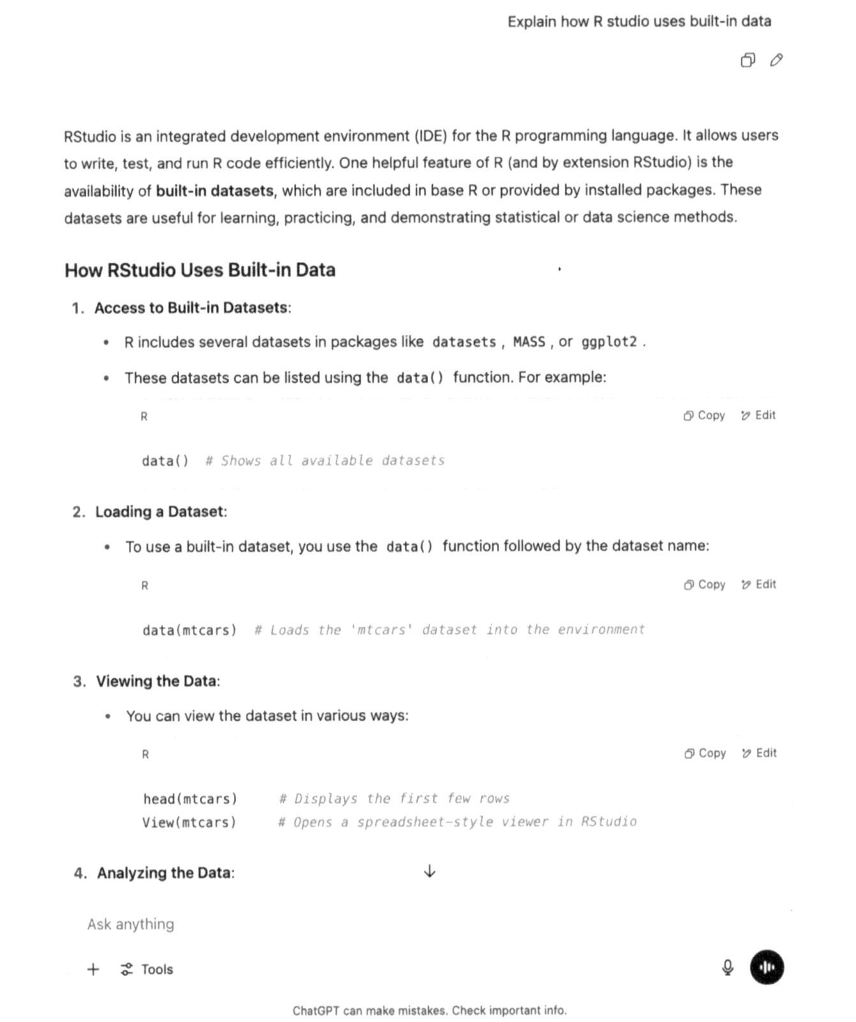

Fig. 3.8 Explanations provided by ChatGPT regarding the use of built-in data in RStudio

As shown in Fig. 3.9, the codes were produced by ChatGPT. The user can copy the codes using the copy function with the icon "copy" located in the upper-right corner of the ChatGPT software interface. The user can then paste (command + v in Mac) the codes in the RStudio software and hit the return key (in Mac) to run the codes in the Console window, as the screenshots of RStudio illustrate in Fig. 3.10:

1. Loading the `iris` Dataset (Built-in)

R Copy Edit

```r
# Load the dataset (already available in base R)
data(iris)

# View the first few rows
head(iris)

# Check the structure
str(iris)
```

2. Loading the `BreastCancer` Dataset (from mlbench package)

R Copy Edit

```r
# Install mlbench package if not already installed
install.packages("mlbench")

# Load the package
library(mlbench)

# Load the dataset
data(BreastCancer)

# View the first few rows
head(BreastCancer)

# Check the structure
str(BreastCancer)
```

Fig. 3.9 Results generated by ChatGPT regarding the use of two RStudio built-in datasets Iris and Breastcancer

External Data

Public health researchers and professionals often rely on external datasets to investigate specific questions. Among these, electronic health records (EHRs) have been increasingly used in research and are valuable for illustrating machine learning (ML) algorithms (Esteva et al., 2019; Rajkomar et al., 2019). In this book, we will utilize a simulated EHR dataset that includes variables of key patient information such as Age, Gender, BMI, Blood Pressure, Heart Rate, Cholesterol Level, Glucose Level, Smoking Status, and Diabetes Status. This dataset will serve as a practical example to demonstrate various ML algorithms.

The dataset is provided as a CSV file on this website. To load and explore the dataset in RStudio, we can use the readr package to import the CSV file. In RStudio,

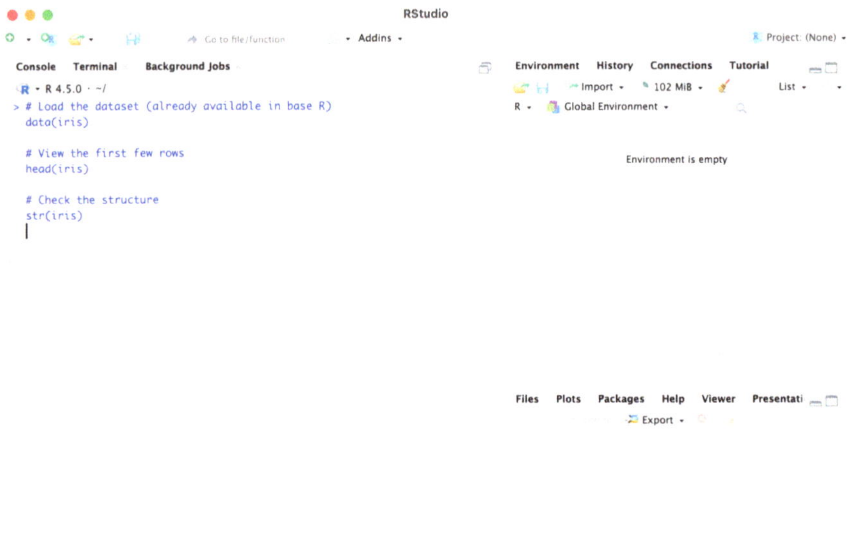

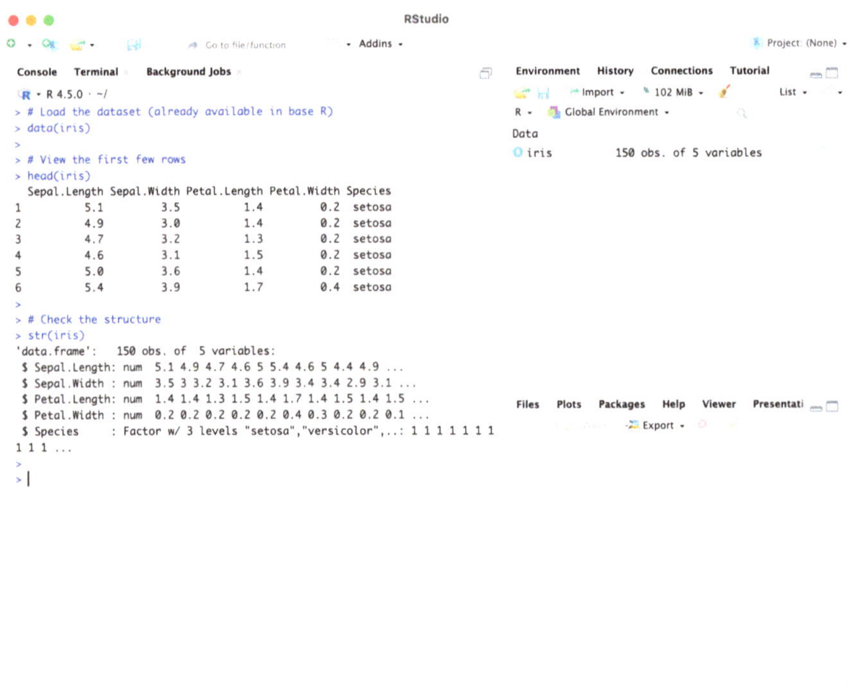

Fig. 3.10 Running the codes generated by ChatGPT in RStudio

Step-by-step Instructions Using `readr`:

r Copy Edit

```r
# Step 1: Install the readr package if not already installed
install.packages("readr")

# Step 2: Load the package
library(readr)

# Step 3: Set your working directory (optional but recommended)
# Example: setwd("/Users/yourname/Documents/yourfolder")

# Step 4: Read the CSV file
ehr_data <- read_csv("simulated_ehr_data_small.csv")

# Step 5: View the first few rows of the dataset
head(ehr_data)

# Step 6: Check the structure of the dataset
str(ehr_data)
```

Fig. 3.11 Step-by-step instructions provided by ChatGPT to use the readr package in RStudio

users should also set the appropriate working directory where the file is saved—this ensures that R can locate the dataset during import.

We can prompt ChatGPT to instruct us how we can upload these external data into RStudio with this prompt: "show how to use the readr package to read an external data called 'simulated_ehr_data_small.csv.'" The results return in ChatGPT as shown in Fig. 3.11:

The R code in Fig. 3.11 demonstrates how to use the `readr` package to import an external dataset named `"simulated_ehr_data_small.csv"` into R. First, the `readr` package is installed and loaded to access the `read_csv()` function, which efficiently reads comma-separated files. The code then assigns the contents of the CSV file to a new object called `ehr_data`. Finally, the `head()` function displays the first few rows of the dataset, and `str()` reveals the structure of the data, including variable types and dimensions. These steps help verify that the dataset has been loaded correctly and is ready for analysis. As shown previously, we can copy the codes and run them in RStudio.

Inspecting the Data

Assuming that the working directory is set correctly, which is where the simulated_ehr_data_small.csv is located, the dataset is now loaded to RStudio. As mentioned, the dataset is now an object assigned as "ehr_data" in RStudio. See Fig. 3.12:

This dataset contains 500 observations and 10 variables, including both numerical and categorical types. For instance, **BMI**, **Blood_Pressure**, and **Heart_Rate** are continuous numerical variables, while **Smoking_Status** and **Diabetes** are categorical. After loading the data in RStudio, users can click on the dataset name (e.g., ehr_data) in the Environment panel to open and view it in a spreadsheet-like format. To explore distributions and relationships between variables, we can use visualization tools such as ggplot2. The codes shown in Fig. 3.13 can be used to visualize the data:

The codes in Fig. 3.13 can be copied and pasted directly into the script editor or console in RStudio and then executed. Once run, the resulting plot will appear in the **Plots** panel, typically located in the lower right section of the RStudio interface. This

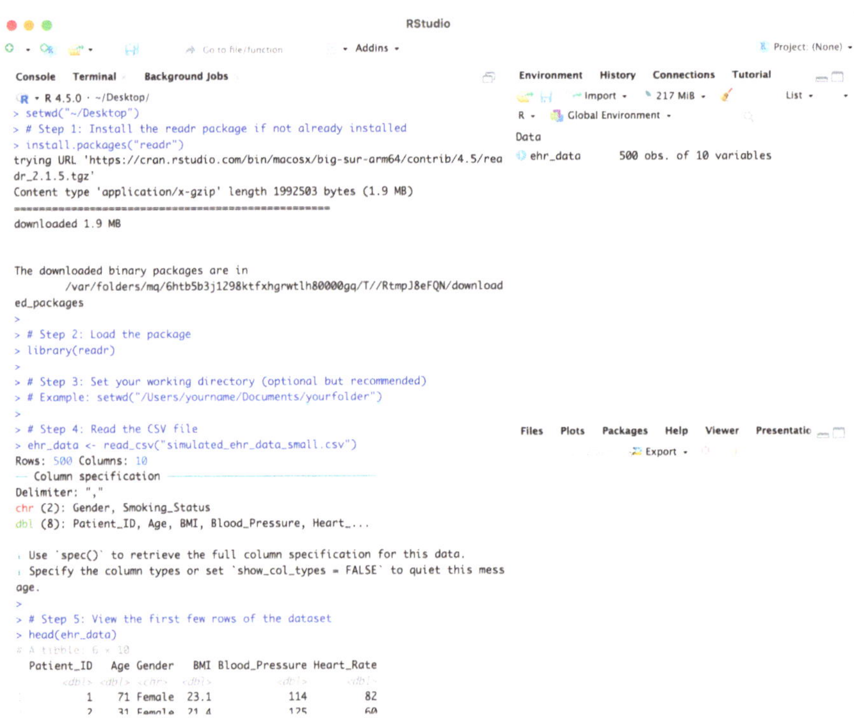

Fig. 3.12 Using RStudio to run the codes generated by ChatGPT to inspect the simulated EHR dataset

Example: Visualizing BMI Distribution

```r
# Load ggplot2 if not already loaded
library(ggplot2)

# Create a histogram of the BMI variable
ggplot(ehr_data, aes(x = BMI)) +
  geom_histogram(binwidth = 2, fill = "steelblue", color = "black") +
  theme_minimal() +
  labs(
    title = "Distribution of BMI in the Simulated EHR Dataset",
    x = "BMI",
    y = "Frequency"
  )
```

Fig. 3.13 R scripts to visualize the distribution of BMI, a variable in the simulated EHR dataset

allows users to visually explore the distribution of variables such as BMI. An example of the output is shown in Fig. 3.14.

To view the graph in a larger window, users can click the **Zoom** button within the Plots panel. This feature is especially helpful for examining details or exporting the plot for presentations and reports. Clicking the Zoom button will return a separate window as shown in Fig. 3.15:

Summary

This chapter introduced R and RStudio as foundational tools for applying machine learning (ML) in public health. It outlined essential steps such as installing R and RStudio, using key packages like caret, ggplot2, and readr, and loading datasets for analysis—including both built-in data (such as iris) and external files (like a simulated EHR dataset).

We also explored how ChatGPT can support learners by assisting with R scripts and clarifying how specific functions and packages work. For example, ChatGPT can generate code to import data, summarize dataset structure, or create visualizations using ggplot2. This guidance helps learners focus on understanding and applying ML techniques rather than struggling with coding issues.

It is important to note that the example prompts provided in this book are not the only ones that will work in ChatGPT. Users can phrase their questions in various ways and still receive helpful results. The key, however, is specificity—the clearer the prompt, the more accurate and useful the response. This flexibility, while

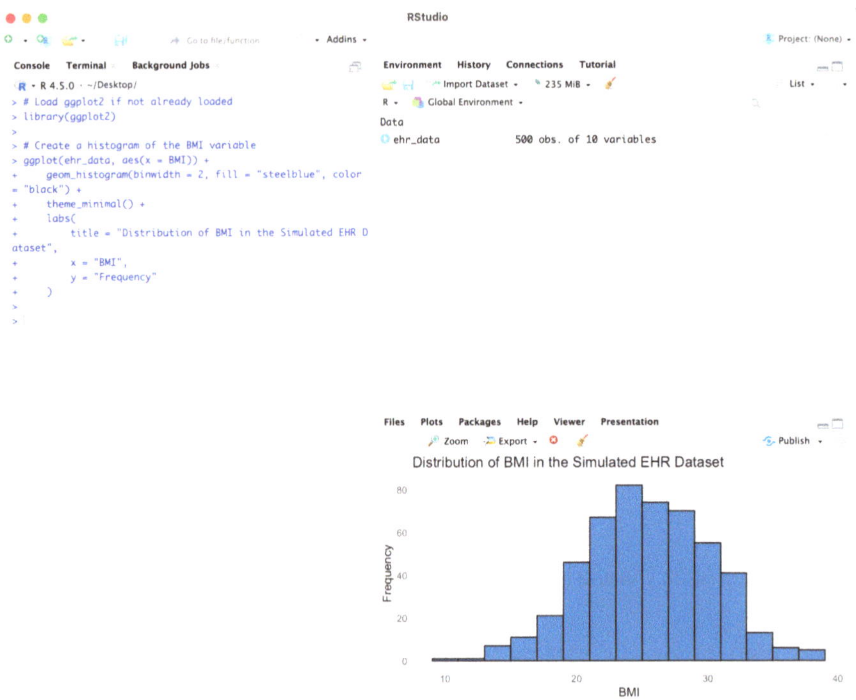

Fig. 3.14 Visualization of the distribution of BMI in RStudio

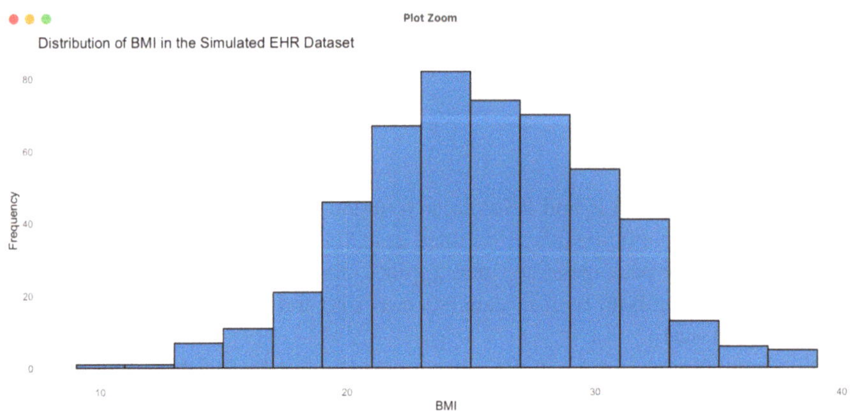

Fig. 3.15 Zooming the visualization of the distribution of BMI in RStudio

beneficial for learning, has also raised concerns about reproducibility. Since similar prompts can produce somewhat different outputs, the use of large language models (LLMs) like ChatGPT in scientific research must be approached thoughtfully. A later chapter will revisit this issue, focusing on how to use GenAI tools responsibly and reproducibly in public health and scientific contexts.

By integrating ChatGPT into their workflow, public health students and professionals can overcome common programming barriers, accelerate their learning process, and more confidently apply data-driven methods to real-world health challenges.

The next chapter (Chap. 4) will introduce **supervised learning**. It will cover core concepts in classification and regression, demonstrate how these algorithms are applied in public health research, and address the ethical considerations involved in their use.

Discussion Questions

1. In what ways do R and RStudio complement each other when conducting public health research, and why is it important to distinguish their roles?
2. What challenges might new users face when installing and configuring R and RStudio for machine learning, and how can these barriers be addressed in educational settings?
3. How can tools like ChatGPT support the learning process in R programming, and what strategies should students use to effectively troubleshoot code or generate scripts?

References

Cunningham, P., Delany, S. J., & Doyle, D. (2021). Machine learning techniques for public health applications: A review. *Computational and Structural Biotechnology Journal, 19*, 4001–4012. https://doi.org/10.1016/j.csbj.2021.06.034

Esteva, A., Robicquet, A., Ramsundar, B., Kuleshov, V., DePristo, M., Chou, K., Cui, C., Corrado, G., Thrun, S., & Dean, J. (2019). A guide to deep learning in healthcare. *Nature Medicine, 25*(1), 24–29. https://doi.org/10.1038/s41591-018-0316-z

Fisher, R. A. (1936). The use of multiple measurements in taxonomic problems. *Annals of Eugenics, 7*(2), 179–188. https://doi.org/10.1111/j.1469-1809.1936.tb02137.x

OpenAI. (n.d.). *ChatGPT*. Retrieved from https://openai.com/chatgpt

R Core Team. (2023). R: A language and environment for statistical computing. R Foundation for Statistical Computing. Retrieved from https://www.r-project.org

Rajkomar, A., Dean, J., & Kohane, I. (2019). Machine learning in medicine. *New England Journal of Medicine, 380*(14), 1347–1358. https://doi.org/10.1056/NEJMra1814259

RStudio, PBC. (2023). RStudio: Integrated development environment for R. Retrieved from https://posit.co

Part II
Machine Learning Techniques and Applications

Chapter 4
Supervised Learning I: Classification Models

Learning Objectives

By the end of this chapter, students will be able to:

1. **Explain** the fundamental concepts of supervised learning.
2. **Apply** classification models to analyze electronic health records (EHR) data.
3. **Evaluate** supervised learning models using appropriate performance metrics.
4. **Use** R and RStudio to prepare, model, and visualize public health data.
5. **Demonstrate** how generative AI (GenAI) tools like ChatGPT can assist in model development, code generation, troubleshooting, and interpretation in supervised ML workflows.

Introduction

Machine learning (ML) is a powerful tool that enables computers to learn patterns from data and make predictions or classifications by automatically identifying relationships in datasets (Samuel, 1959). In public health, ML can be used to identify disease risks, predict patient outcomes, and improve decision-making in healthcare (Esteva et al., 2017; Rajkomar et al., 2019).

For example, ML can help predict the likelihood of hospital readmission based on patient demographics and medical history (Leung et al., 2017). Research has shown promising results in using machine learning algorithms to analyze electronic health records and identify patients at high risk for readmission. Another application is in epidemiology, where ML can classify whether an individual is at high or low risk for developing diabetes based on lifestyle and genetic factors (Xie et al., 2019). These

---

Supplementary Information The online version contains supplementary material available at https://doi.org/10.1007/978-3-032-08677-8_4.

R. Leung, *Leveraging GenAI for Machine Learning Education in Public Health*,
https://doi.org/10.1007/978-3-032-08677-8_4

models assist healthcare professionals by providing data-driven insights that improve patient care and resource allocation.

A key aspect of ML is how data are used during model development. Unlike traditional statistical analysis, where all available data are used at once to maximize sample size, ML partitions data into training and testing sets (Goodfellow et al., 2016). The training data are used to develop the model, while the testing data evaluate its predictive accuracy. More advanced ML workflows may also use validation data to fine-tune the model before final testing. This approach ensures that the model generalizes well to new, unseen data rather than simply memorizing patterns from the training data. In this sense, ML "recycles" data by dividing the same dataset into separate phases to test and improve predictive performance.

Supervised Learning

Supervised learning represents one of the fundamental approaches in machine learning, characterized by its use of labeled training data to teach algorithms how to make predictions on new, unseen data. This paradigm encompasses two distinct but complementary methodologies that address different types of prediction problems in public health applications. Before diving into theoretical foundations, we will begin with a quick demonstration showing how these models can be rapidly implemented in RStudio, either through direct coding or with assistance from artificial intelligence (AI) tools like ChatGPT to generate the necessary R code.

Classification tasks focus on predicting discrete outcomes or categorical labels from input data. In healthcare contexts, classification algorithms excel at diagnostic applications where clear categorical distinctions are essential. For example, medical imaging analysis systems can distinguish between benign and malignant tumors by learning patterns from thousands of previously diagnosed cases (Esteva et al., 2019). Similarly, classification models can predict whether patients are at high, medium, or low risk for developing specific conditions based on their demographic and clinical profiles.

Regression analysis, in contrast, addresses problems requiring continuous numerical predictions. These models prove particularly valuable when healthcare professionals need precise quantitative estimates rather than categorical classifications. Blood pressure prediction systems exemplify this approach, using current health indicators such as age, weight, exercise habits, and existing medical conditions to forecast future cardiovascular measurements (Rajkomar et al., 2019). Regression techniques also support resource planning by predicting hospital admission rates, treatment costs, and recovery timeframes.

The following sections will introduce four essential supervised learning algorithms: k-nearest neighbors (KNN), logistic regression, decision trees, and random forest models. To facilitate understanding of these fundamental techniques, we will demonstrate their implementation using built-in R datasets that provide clear, accessible examples of each algorithm's strengths and applications. These foundational concepts will serve as preparation for a later chapter, where we will revisit and apply these same modeling approaches to authentic electronic health record (EHR) data, illustrating how these techniques translate to complex, real-world healthcare analytics scenarios. While the initial demonstrations will focus on quickly running these models to show their basic functionality, subsequent sections will provide comprehensive details about each algorithm's underlying mechanics, parameter tuning, and appropriate evaluative metrics.

Training and Test Data in Supervised Learning

A fundamental principle of supervised machine learning is dividing the available dataset into training and test subsets. This practice is essential for developing reliable predictive models and ensuring that model evaluation reflects real-world performance rather than simply measuring how well the model "remembers" the training data.

Why Use Training and Test Data?

- **Training data** is used to "teach" the algorithm by exposing it to examples with known outcomes (labels). The model identifies patterns and learns the relationship between predictor variables (e.g., age, blood pressure) and outcomes (e.g., disease status).
- **Test data** is set aside and not used during training. Instead, it is reserved for objectively evaluating the model's predictive ability on new, unseen data. This process helps detect overfitting—where a model performs well on training data but fails to generalize to new cases.

Importance in Classification Models

For classification models, such as those used to predict binary or multiclass outcomes (e.g., disease presence, survival, or risk group), splitting data into training and test sets ensures that the model's classification accuracy and other performance metrics (e.g., sensitivity, specificity, confusion matrix) are valid and not biased by prior exposure to the answers.

Common Practice Across ML Models

The approach of splitting data is common to all four classification models illustrated in this text—K-Nearest Neighbors (KNN), logistic regression, decision tree, and random forest. Regardless of the model's complexity or underlying methodology, all require an unbiased test of predictive performance. This ensures fair model comparison and supports trustworthy deployment in public health or management settings.

R Code for Data Splitting

In R, data splitting is commonly performed using the caret package and its createDataPartition() function. We can ask ChatGPT to provide a sample R code for data splitting by using the prompt such as "show how R split training and test data." The results are shown in Fig. 4.1:

Note that the R code provided above for data splitting will only work if the **`caret`** package is properly installed and loaded in your R or RStudio environment. This is also true for other R packages referenced in this book—each must be installed before use, typically via the `install.packages()` function. Figure 4.2 illustrates how the R code appears when executed within the RStudio interface, highlighting the installation of the caret package, coding environment and output display.

K-Nearest Neighbors (KNN)

The K-Nearest Neighbors (KNN) algorithm is intuitive and applicable in public health scenarios, such as classifying patients into risk groups based on clinical features. The KNN algorithm classifies new observations based on their proximity to existing labeled data points. Specifically, it identifies the "k" closest observations (neighbors) from the training dataset to the new data point, then assigns the class that appears most frequently among these neighbors. KNN is straightforward as it requires minimal assumptions about the underlying data distribution, making it robust for diverse public health datasets. The effectiveness of KNN depends significantly on selecting an optimal number of neighbors ("k"), typically determined through cross-validation or other performance evaluation methods.

The KNN algorithm computes distance using the Euclidean metric, defined as:

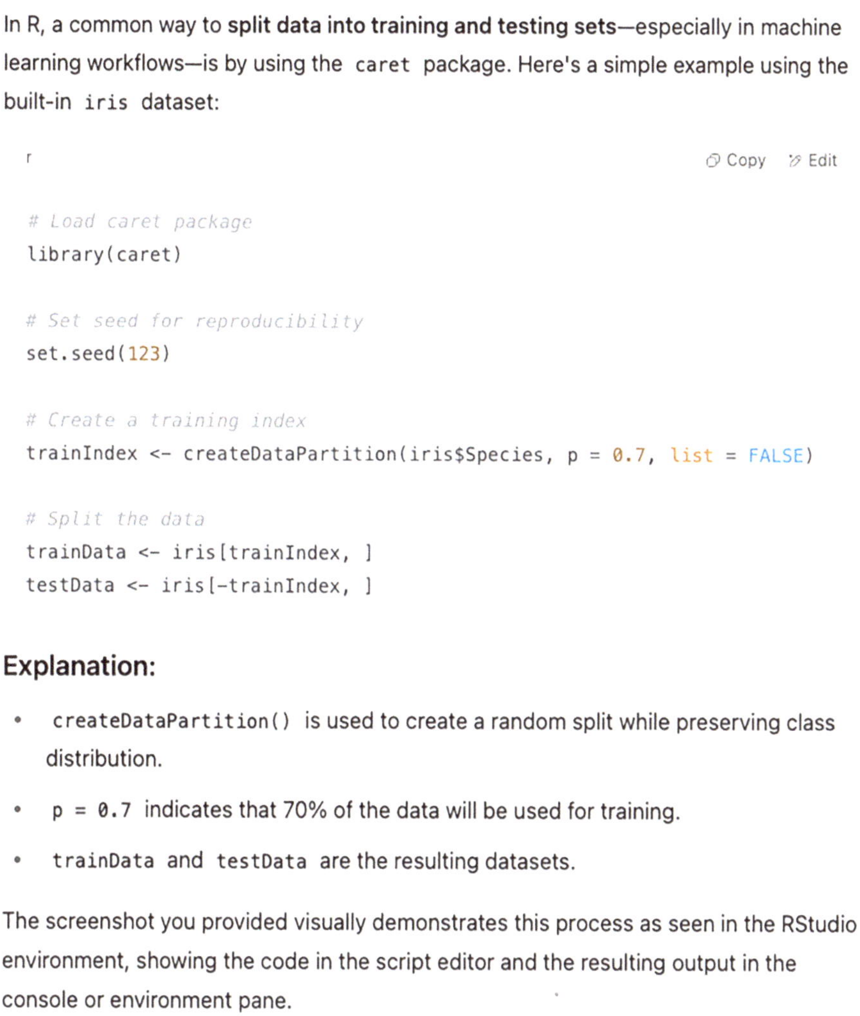

In R, a common way to **split data into training and testing sets**—especially in machine learning workflows—is by using the `caret` package. Here's a simple example using the built-in `iris` dataset:

r Copy Edit

```
# Load caret package
library(caret)

# Set seed for reproducibility
set.seed(123)

# Create a training index
trainIndex <- createDataPartition(iris$Species, p = 0.7, list = FALSE)

# Split the data
trainData <- iris[trainIndex, ]
testData <- iris[-trainIndex, ]
```

Explanation:

- `createDataPartition()` is used to create a random split while preserving class distribution.
- `p = 0.7` indicates that 70% of the data will be used for training.
- `trainData` and `testData` are the resulting datasets.

The screenshot you provided visually demonstrates this process as seen in the RStudio environment, showing the code in the script editor and the resulting output in the console or environment pane.

Fig. 4.1 Data partition steps generated by ChatGPT for supervised learning

$$d(x,y) = \sqrt{\sum_{i=1}^{n} (x_i - y_i)^2}$$

where:

- $d(x, y)$ is the Euclidean distance between observations x and y,
- x_i and y_i represent the respective values of feature i in the observations,
- n is the number of features.

The observations with the smallest distances to the new data point are selected as its nearest neighbors.

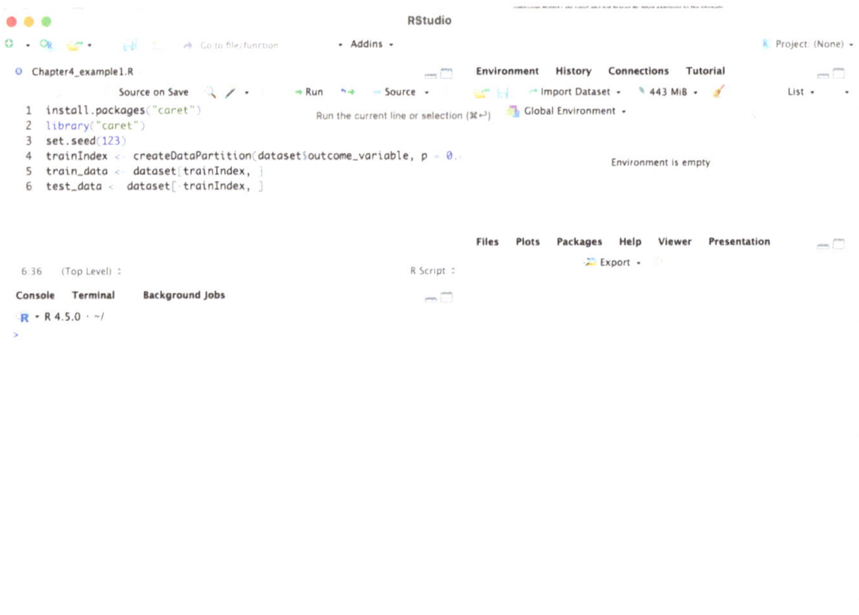

Fig. 4.2 Data partition steps executed in RStudio

Iris Dataset Example

To illustrate KNN clearly, we use the built-in R dataset **iris**. The iris dataset contains measurements for three species of iris flowers: *setosa*, *versicolor*, and *virginica*. The dataset features four predictor variables (sepal length, sepal width, petal length, and petal width), making it ideal for demonstrating classification techniques. ChatGPT can significantly streamline the process of implementing KNN in R by providing clear, tailored code. Users can prompt ChatGPT with specific questions, such as:

"Provide R code to apply KNN classification on the iris dataset, including splitting the data, normalization, and evaluating accuracy." Based on this prompt, ChatGPT generates the example code as shown in Fig. 4.3:

The R code generated by ChatGPT (see Fig. 4.3) demonstrates the process of applying the KNN classification algorithm using the iris dataset. It involves several essential steps: loading necessary libraries, importing and splitting the dataset into training and testing subsets, normalizing the predictor variables for consistent scale, implementing the KNN classification, and finally evaluating model performance through a confusion matrix. This workflow is structured to enhance clarity, reproducibility, and ease of interpretation, making it particularly useful for public health professionals developing classification models for clinical or epidemiological decision-making.

R Copy Edit

```
# Load necessary libraries
library(caret)
library(class)

# Load iris dataset
data(iris)

# Set random seed for reproducibility
set.seed(123)

# Split data into training (80%) and test (20%) sets
trainIndex <- createDataPartition(iris$Species, p = 0.8, list = FALSE)
train_data <- iris[trainIndex,]
test_data <- iris[-trainIndex,]

# Normalize predictor variables
preProcValues <- preProcess(train_data[, 1:4], method = c("center", "scale"))
train_data_norm <- predict(preProcValues, train_data[, 1:4])
test_data_norm <- predict(preProcValues, test_data[, 1:4])

# Apply KNN classification (k=5)
knn_predictions <- knn(train = train_data_norm,
                       test = test_data_norm,
                       cl = train_data$Species,
                       k = 5)

# Evaluate model accuracy
conf_matrix <- confusionMatrix(knn_predictions, test_data$Species)
print(conf_matrix)
```

Fig. 4.3 R code generated by ChatGPT to perform the KNN algorithm

We can ask ChatGPT to explain in greater detail what the above codes accomplish by using a prompt such as "provide explanations about what the codes were doing in RStudio." The following results return (see Fig. 4.4):

Following the iris example as shown in Figs. 4.3 and 4.4 the K-Nearest Neighbors (KNN) algorithm can similarly be applied to Electronic Health Records (EHR) to classify patients into **high, medium, or low risk** categories for diabetes based on their clinical features. With EHR data, KNN identifies existing patients whose profiles—such as age, cholesterol levels, blood pressure, BMI, and glucose levels—are most similar to a new patient. The algorithm then assigns a risk level based on the most common category among the nearest neighbors. For example, if most similar patients were categorized as high risk, the new patient would be classified accordingly. Because KNN uses direct comparisons rather than complex model

Explanation of KNN Classification Code in RStudio

1. Load Necessary Libraries

R Copy Edit

```r
library(caret)
library(class)
```

- `caret` : Provides functions for training and evaluating machine learning models, including splitting datasets and preprocessing.
- `class` : Contains the `knn()` function specifically for implementing K-Nearest Neighbors classification.

2. Load the Iris Dataset

R Copy Edit

```r
data(iris)
```

- The `data()` function loads built-in datasets from R packages. Here, `iris` dataset is loaded, containing flower measurements for three iris species.

3. Splitting the Data into Training and Test Sets

R Copy Edit

```r
set.seed(123)
trainIndex <- createDataPartition(iris$Species, p = 0.8, list = FALSE)
train_data <- iris[trainIndex,]
test_data <- iris[-trainIndex,]
```

- `set.seed(123)` : Ensures reproducibility by setting a fixed random seed.
- `createDataPartition()` : Splits the data into training (80%) and test (20%) sets, ensuring each subset is representative of the original data distribution.
- `train_data` and `test_data` : These subsets are essential for training the KNN model and evaluating its accuracy, respectively.

Fig. 4.4 Explanations generated by ChatGPT to explain how the KNN algorithm is performed in RStudio

assumptions, it is well-suited for analyzing diverse and heterogeneous clinical data. This makes it an accessible and interpretable method for informing population health strategies, guiding early interventions, and supporting individualized diabetes prevention in public health practice.

4. Normalizing Predictor Variables

R

Copy Edit

```
preProcValues <- preProcess(train_data[, 1:4], method = c("center", "scale"))
train_data_norm <- predict(preProcValues, train_data[, 1:4])
test_data_norm <- predict(preProcValues, test_data[, 1:4])
```

- Normalization is crucial because KNN is sensitive to feature scale differences.
- `preProcess()` : Calculates parameters (mean and standard deviation) from the training dataset used to standardize (center and scale) the predictor variables.
- `predict(preProcValues, ...)` : Applies the calculated normalization parameters to both training and test sets, ensuring consistent scaling.

5. Applying KNN Classification

R

Copy Edit

```
knn_predictions <- knn(train = train_data_norm,
                       test = test_data_norm,
                       cl = train_data$Species,
                       k = 5)
```

- `knn()` function classifies test observations based on their proximity to training observations.
- Arguments:
  - `train` : Normalized training data.
  - `test` : Normalized test data.
  - `cl` : Known labels from training data.
  - `k` : The number of nearest neighbors used to make the classification decision (here, k=5).

6. Evaluating Model Accuracy

R

Copy Edit

```
conf_matrix <- confusionMatrix(knn_predictions, test_data$Species)
print(conf_matrix)
```

- `confusionMatrix()` : Compares predicted species with actual species, providing accuracy metrics, sensitivity, specificity, and a detailed confusion matrix.
- `print(conf_matrix)` : Displays the detailed evaluation metrics clearly in RStudio, helping users assess model performance.

Fig. 4.4 (continued)

Logistic Regression

Logistic regression is another **classification model** commonly used in supervised learning to predict binary outcomes. In public health, it helps estimate the probability of a patient having a particular condition (e.g., diabetes: yes/no) based on a set of predictor variables such as age, BMI, or lab results (Hosmer et al., 2013). Logistic regression outputs probabilities between 0 and 1, making it useful for risk prediction and decision-making in clinical and epidemiological contexts. Typically, predicted probabilities of 0.5 or higher will be classified as "1" or positive. Predicted probabilities lower than 0.5 are classified as "0" or negative. The 0.5 threshold is adjustable based on the specific clinical context and the relative costs of false positives versus false negatives.

The logistic regression formula is shown as follows:

$$P(Y = 1 \mid X) = \frac{1}{1 + e^{-(\beta_0 + \beta_1 X_1 + \beta_2 X_2 + \cdots + \beta_n X_n)}}$$

where:

- $P(Y = 1|X)$: Probability that the outcome Y equals 1, given predictors (also called features in ML) X_1, X_2, …, X_n.
- β_0: Intercept (baseline log-odds)
- $\beta_1, \beta_2, \ldots, \beta_n$: Coefficients for the predictor variables (also called features in ML)
- $X_1, X_2, \ldots, X_n$: Predictor variables (also called features in ML)(e.g., age, BMI, cholesterol)

The equation uses the logistic (sigmoid) function to transform a linear combination of predictors into a probability between 0 and 1. In classification tasks, the predicted probability is then used to assign as outcome class, such as:

- If $P(Y = 1 \mid X) \geq 0.5$, classify the observation as "1" (positive class, e.g., disease present).
- If $P(Y = 1 \mid X) < 0.5$, classify the observation as "0" (negative class, e.g., disease absent).

The threshold (commonly 0.5) can be adjusted depending on the context and cost of false positives vs. false negatives, which can be very important in public health applications like disease screening or risk assessment.

Mtcars Data Example

To illustrate the practical application of logistic regression, we will utilize the built-in **mtcars** dataset within RStudio. Although this dataset originates from the automotive domain, it provides an excellent pedagogical framework for understanding logistic regression methodology before applying these techniques to health data. In this demonstration, we will model the binary variable am (0 = automatic transmission, 1 = manual transmission) as our outcome variable and examine how predictor variables such as mpg (miles per gallon), hp (horsepower), and wt (weight) function as features to predict our target outcome—transmission type. This analytical framework directly parallels health-related logistic regression applications, where binary health outcomes (such as disease presence/absence) are predicted using continuous clinical variables (such as biomarkers, vital signs, or demographic factors). The structural similarity between predicting transmission type from car characteristics and predicting health outcomes from patient characteristics makes this an ideal introductory example for understanding the logistic regression process.

To illustrate logistic regression clearly, we use the built-in R dataset `mtcars`. Although originally developed for automotive performance analysis, the dataset is frequently used in data science education due to its clean structure and binary variables. In this case, we model the variable `am` (0 = automatic, 1 = manual transmission) as the binary outcome. The predictors include continuous variables such as miles per gallon (`mpg`), horsepower (`hp`), and vehicle weight (`wt`), which are analogous to continuous clinical indicators in a public health context (e.g., BMI, blood pressure, cholesterol).

ChatGPT can significantly streamline the process of implementing logistic regression in R by generating clear, step-by-step code. Users can prompt ChatGPT with a question like: "Provide R code to apply logistic regression on the mtcars dataset, including model fitting and interpretation of output."

Based on this prompt, ChatGPT generates the example code shown in Fig. 4.5:

The R code generated by ChatGPT demonstrates the process of applying the **logistic regression** classification algorithm using the `mtcars` dataset. It follows a structured workflow that includes loading necessary libraries, converting the binary outcome variable (`am`) to a factor, splitting the data into training and testing sets, fitting a logistic regression model using selected predictor variables (`mpg`, `hp.`, and `wt`), and evaluating model performance through predicted probabilities, binary classification, and a confusion matrix. This process ensures reproducibility, interpretability, and practical relevance—particularly for public health professionals seeking to develop risk prediction models for binary outcomes such as disease presence or treatment response.

We can also ask ChatGPT to explain what the above code accomplishes by using a prompt such as: "Provide explanations about what the logistic regression code was doing in RStudio."

ChatGPT would then return detailed, step-by-step interpretations of each line of code to support learning and application. The following results return (see Fig. 4.6):

Following the mtcars example above, **logistic regression** can similarly be applied to electronic health records (EHR) to predict the likelihood that a patient is at risk for **cardiovascular disease**. Using clinical features such as age, BMI, blood pressure, cholesterol levels, and heart rate as predictors, logistic regression estimates the probability of a binary outcome—such as whether a patient has or is likely to develop cardiovascular disease (yes/no). Based on a predefined threshold

```r
# Load necessary libraries
library(caret)      # for data splitting and evaluation
library(dplyr)      # for data manipulation

# Load the dataset
data(mtcars)

# Convert outcome variable to factor (am: 0 = automatic, 1 = manual)
mtcars$am <- as.factor(mtcars$am)

# Set seed for reproducibility
set.seed(123)

# Split the dataset into training (80%) and testing (20%)
trainIndex <- createDataPartition(mtcars$am, p = 0.8, list = FALSE)
train_data <- mtcars[trainIndex, ]
test_data <- mtcars[-trainIndex, ]

# Fit logistic regression model
logit_model <- glm(am ~ mpg + hp + wt, data = train_data, family = binomial)

# Summary of the model (interpretation)
summary(logit_model)

# Predict probabilities on the test set
pred_probs <- predict(logit_model, newdata = test_data, type = "response")

# Convert probabilities to binary class using 0.5 threshold
pred_class <- ifelse(pred_probs > 0.5, 1, 0)
pred_class <- as.factor(pred_class)

# Confusion matrix and accuracy
conf_matrix <- confusionMatrix(pred_class, test_data$am)
print(conf_matrix)
```

Fig. 4.5 R code generated by ChatGPT to perform the logistic regression algorithm

(commonly 0.5), the model classifies patients into outcome categories. For example, if a patient's predicted probability equals or exceeds 0.5, they may be flagged as high risk for cardiovascular disease. This method also provides interpretable coefficients (odds ratios), helping public health professionals understand which factors most strongly contribute to cardiovascular risk. As a result, logistic regression serves as a practical and transparent tool for identifying at-risk individuals, guiding clinical decision-making, and supporting population-level prevention strategies.

1. Load Necessary Libraries

r Copy Edit

```r
library(caret)
library(dplyr)
```

- `caret` : Used for data splitting and model evaluation.
- `dplyr` : Provides data manipulation tools.

2. Load the Dataset

r Copy Edit

```r
data(mtcars)
```

- Loads the built-in `mtcars` dataset, which contains 32 observations on 11 variables related to automobile design and performance.

3. Convert the Outcome Variable to a Factor

r Copy Edit

```r
mtcars$am <- as.factor(mtcars$am)
```

- Converts the binary outcome variable `am` (0 = automatic, 1 = manual) to a factor so it can be used as a categorical dependent variable in logistic regression.

Fig. 4.6 Explanations generated by ChatGPT regarding how the logistic regression algorithm is performed in RStudio

Decision Tree

Decision tree (DT) is a versatile classification and regression model commonly used in supervised learning to predict both binary and multiclass outcomes. In public health, decision trees help identify patterns and decision rules for patient classification (e.g., high/medium/low risk categories) based on a set of predictor variables such as age, symptoms, or diagnostic test results (Breiman et al., 1984). Decision trees create a flowchart-like structure that splits data based on feature values, making them highly interpretable for clinical decision-making. Each internal node represents a test on a feature, each branch represents the outcome of the test, and each leaf node

4. Split the Data into Training and Test Sets

r Copy Edit

```r
set.seed(123)
trainIndex <- createDataPartition(mtcars$am, p = 0.8, list = FALSE)
train_data <- mtcars[trainIndex, ]
test_data <- mtcars[-trainIndex, ]
```

- `set.seed(123)` : Ensures reproducibility of random splits.
- `createDataPartition()` : Splits the data into 80% training and 20% testing subsets.
- `train_data` and `test_data` : Used to fit the model and evaluate performance, respectively.

5. Fit the Logistic Regression Model

r Copy Edit

```r
logit_model <- glm(am ~ mpg + hp + wt, data = train_data, family = binomial)
```

- `glm()` : Fits a generalized linear model.
- `am ~ mpg + hp + wt` : Models transmission type based on fuel efficiency (`mpg`), horsepower (`hp`), and weight (`wt`).
- `family = binomial` : Specifies logistic regression for binary outcomes.

6. Display Model Summary

r Copy Edit

```r
summary(logit_model)
```

- Provides coefficient estimates, standard errors, z-values, and p-values.
- Helps interpret how each predictor influences the odds of manual vs. automatic transmission.

Fig. 4.6 (continued)

represents a class prediction or decision outcome. The model's transparency allows healthcare professionals to understand exactly how predictions are made, which is crucial for clinical applications.

7. Predict Probabilities on the Test Set

r Copy Edit

```r
pred_probs <- predict(logit_model, newdata = test_data, type = "response")
```

- Generates predicted probabilities for the test set.
- `type = "response"` : Ensures predictions are returned as probabilities between 0 and 1.

8. Convert Probabilities to Binary Predictions

r Copy Edit

```r
pred_class <- ifelse(pred_probs > 0.5, 1, 0)
pred_class <- as.factor(pred_class)
```

- Converts probabilities to binary class predictions using a threshold of 0.5.
- Probabilities ≥ 0.5 are classified as `1` (manual), and < 0.5 as `0` (automatic).

9. Evaluate Model Performance

r Copy Edit

```r
conf_matrix <- confusionMatrix(pred_class, test_data$am)
print(conf_matrix)
```

- `confusionMatrix()` : Compares predicted classes to actual test set labels.
- Outputs accuracy, sensitivity, specificity, and a full confusion matrix to assess how well the model performs.

Fig. 4.6 (continued)

Unlike regression or logistic regression, decision trees do not use a single algebraic formula for prediction. Instead, a decision tree model is built through a recursive process that splits the dataset into subsets using decision rules based on feature values. However, the key idea behind a decision tree split is straightforward. All the data constitute the root node of the decision tree to be generated by the algorithm. Starting from the root node, and at each subsequent node, the DT algorithm selects a specific value of a particular feature that maximizes the separation between classes, commonly using criteria such as Gini impurity or information gain (also called entropy). For example, if the selected split at a node was bass mass index (BMI) < 20, the data would be divided into a class with all observations (e.g., patients) that had a BMI value of under 20, and a class with all observations that had a BMI value of 20 or above. In this example, the "BMI $<$ 20" was selected because either the Gini impurity or the information gain criterion was fulfilled.

Once the data is split at a parent node, two child nodes are created. The child nodes may or may not be further split, depending on the algorithm. Mathematically, the two criteria Gina impurity and information gain (or entropy) may be represented as follows:

Gini Impurity (for Classification Trees)

$$Gini(t) = 1 - \sum_{i=1}^{C} p_i^2$$

where:

- t = node of the tree
- C = number of classes
- p_i= proportion of samples belonging to class i at node t

Information Gain

$$Entropy(t) = -\sum_{i=1}^{C} p_i \log_2 p_i$$

$$\text{Information Gain} = Entropy(parent) - \sum_{j=1}^{k} \frac{N_j}{N} \cdot Entropy(j)$$

where:

- N = total samples at parent node
- N_j = samples at child node j.
- k = number of child nodes after the split.

A decision tree model predicts outcomes by following a series of logical "if–then" rules determined by splits that maximize purity (reduce impurity) according to a chosen criterion (such as Gini impurity or entropy). There is no simple linear formula; instead, the tree structure itself encodes the prediction process.

Titanic Data Example

To illustrate the practical application of decision trees, we will utilize the built-in **Titanic** dataset within RStudio. Originally compiled from historical records of the RMS Titanic disaster, this dataset provides an excellent pedagogical framework for understanding decision tree methodology before applying these techniques to health data. The dataset is frequently used in data science education due to its mix of categorical and continuous variables with a clear binary outcome. In this demonstration, we will model the binary variable Survived (No = died, Yes = survived) as our outcome variable and examine how predictor variables such as Class (passenger class), Sex, and Age function as features to predict our target outcome—passenger survival. The predictors include both categorical variables such as passenger class and sex, and continuous variables such as age, which are analogous to the mixed-type clinical indicators commonly found in public health contexts (e.g., demographic categories, socioeconomic factors, and continuous biomarkers).

This analytical framework directly parallels health-related decision tree applications, where binary health outcomes (such as treatment success/failure or disease presence/absence) are predicted using mixed-type clinical variables. The structural similarity between predicting survival from passenger characteristics and predicting health outcomes from patient characteristics makes this an ideal introductory example for understanding the decision tree process.

ChatGPT can significantly streamline the process of implementing decision trees in R by generating clear, step-by-step code. Users can prompt ChatGPT with a question like: "Provide R code to apply decision tree classification on the Titanic dataset, including model fitting, visualization, and interpretation of output."

Based on this prompt, ChatGPT generates the example code shown in Fig. 4.7:

The R code generated by ChatGPT demonstrates the process of applying the decision tree classification algorithm using the Titanic dataset. It follows a structured workflow that includes loading the necessary libraries, selecting and cleaning relevant variables (such as Survived, Pclass, Sex, and Age), splitting the data into training and testing sets, fitting a decision tree model using selected predictors, and evaluating model performance with predictions and a confusion matrix. This process ensures reproducibility, interpretability, and practical relevance—particularly for public health professionals seeking to develop transparent and actionable risk prediction tools for binary outcomes such as survival or disease status.

We can also ask ChatGPT to explain what the above code accomplishes by using a prompt such as: "Provide explanations about what the decision tree code was doing in RStudio." ChatGPT would then return detailed, step-by-step interpretations of each line of code to support learning and application. The following results return (see Fig. 4.8):

Following the Titanic example above, the DT algorithm can also be applied to electronic health records (EHR) to classify patients according to their risk of cardiovascular disease. Using clinical features such as age, BMI, blood pressure, cholesterol levels, and heart rate as input variables, a decision tree model recursively

r Copy Edit

```r
# ============================================================
# Decision Tree with Titanic Data Example (Fixed)
# ============================================================

# Install and load packages if needed
# install.packages("titanic")
library(titanic)
library(rpart)      # for decision tree
library(rpart.plot) # for plotting
library(caret)      # for train/test split and evaluation
library(dplyr)

# Prepare dataset (select relevant columns and remove NAs)
titanic_data <- titanic_train %>%
  select(Survived, Pclass, Sex, Age, SibSp, Parch, Fare, Embarked) %>%
  na.omit()

# Convert variables to factors where appropriate
titanic_data$Survived <- as.factor(titanic_data$Survived)
titanic_data$Pclass   <- as.factor(titanic_data$Pclass)
titanic_data$Sex      <- as.factor(titanic_data$Sex)
titanic_data$Embarked <- as.factor(titanic_data$Embarked)

# Split into training and testing sets (80/20)
set.seed(123)
trainIndex <- createDataPartition(titanic_data$Survived, p = 0.8, list = FALSE)
train_data <- titanic_data[trainIndex, ]
test_data  <- titanic_data[-trainIndex, ]

# Ensure Survived in test_data has the same factor levels as in train_data
test_data$Survived <- factor(test_data$Survived, levels = levels(train_data$Survived))

# Fit decision tree model
tree_model <- rpart(Survived ~ Pclass + Sex + Age, data = train_data, method = "class")

# Visualize the decision tree
rpart.plot(tree_model)

# Predict on test data
tree_preds <- predict(tree_model, test_data, type = "class")

# Ensure predictions are factors with same levels as reference
tree_preds <- factor(tree_preds, levels = levels(test_data$Survived))

# Confusion matrix
confusionMatrix(tree_preds, test_data$Survived)
```

Fig. 4.7 R code generated by ChatGPT regarding how the decision tree algorithm is performed in RStudio

1) Load packages

- `titanic` : provides the sample Titanic dataset.
- `rpart` : fits the decision tree (CART) model.
- `rpart.plot` : plots the fitted tree with readable node labels.
- `caret` : convenient utilities for splitting data and evaluating models.
- `dplyr` : data wrangling (selecting variables, handling missing values).

Why it matters: These libraries give you a complete pipeline—from data prep to modeling to interpretation —common in analytics projects.

2) Prepare the dataset

r   Copy   Edit

```r
titanic_data <- titanic_train %>%
  select(Survived, Pclass, Sex, Age, SibSp, Parch, Fare, Embarked) %>%
  na.omit()
```

- Keeps the outcome (`Survived`) and relevant predictors.
- Removes rows with missing values for a clean example.

Why it matters: Clear variable selection and handling missingness reduce noise and make results reproducible.

3) Convert types (factors vs. numeric)

r   Copy   Edit

```r
titanic_data$Survived <- as.factor(titanic_data$Survived)
titanic_data$Pclass   <- as.factor(titanic_data$Pclass)
titanic_data$Sex      <- as.factor(titanic_data$Sex)
titanic_data$Embarked <- as.factor(titanic_data$Embarked)
```

- Tells R which variables are categorical.
- The outcome `Survived` must be a factor for classification.

Why it matters: Trees treat numeric and categorical predictors differently; correct typing avoids errors and improves model quality.

4) Split into training and testing sets

r   Copy   Edit

```r
set.seed(123)
trainIndex <- createDataPartition(titanic_data$Survived, p = 0.8, list = FALSE)
train_data <- titanic_data[trainIndex, ]
test_data  <- titanic_data[-trainIndex, ]
```

- Uses stratified sampling so class proportions are similar in train/test.
- `set.seed()` ensures reproducibility.

Why it matters: A hold-out test set provides an honest estimate of real-world performance—standard practice in analytics.

Fig. 4.8 Explanations generated by ChatGPT regarding how the decision tree algorithm is performed in RStudio

5) Fit the decision tree

r Copy Edit

```r
tree_model <- rpart(Survived ~ Pclass + Sex + Age, data = train_data, method = "class")
```

- CART algorithm recursively splits the data to maximize class purity (e.g., Gini index).
- Uses three predictors for clarity; you can add others.

What the model learns: Simple if-then rules (e.g., "If Sex = female then …") that segment passengers into groups with different survival probabilities—easy to communicate to non-technical stakeholders.

6) Visualize the tree

r Copy Edit

```r
rpart.plot(tree_model, type = 2, extra = 104, fallen.leaves = TRUE)
```

- Draws a labeled tree.
- Nodes display predicted class, class probabilities, and sample sizes.

Why it matters: The plot shows decision logic transparently (interpretability is a key advantage of trees in management settings).

7) Generate predictions on the test set

r Copy Edit

```r
tree_preds <- predict(tree_model, newdata = test_data, type = "class")
```

- Produces predicted classes ("0/1" or "No/Yes" depending on factor levels).

8) Evaluate performance

r Copy Edit

```r
confusionMatrix(tree_preds, test_data$Survived)
```

- Compares predictions to actual outcomes.
- Reports accuracy, sensitivity (recall for the positive class), specificity, and more.

Why it matters: These metrics quantify how well the rules would generalize to new cases—supporting evidence-based decisions.

Fig. 4.8 (continued)

splits the patient data into branches based on threshold values that best separate groups with different risk profiles. This process results in a clear, interpretable set of decision rules, where each pathway through the tree leads to a specific risk classification (such as high or low risk for cardiovascular disease). The visual structure of a decision tree helps public health professionals and clinicians quickly identify which factors and cutoff values most strongly influence risk, supporting transparent and data-driven decision-making. As a result, decision tree models are valuable tools for individualized risk assessment, clinical screening, and population health planning.

Random Forest

Random forest is an advanced ensemble learning method and a direct extension of the decision tree model. It builds multiple decision trees on bootstrapped subsets of the data and aggregates their predictions to produce a final classification or regression outcome (Breiman, 2001). In public health, random forests are especially useful for complex prediction tasks where individual risk profiles must be identified from a large set of variables—such as demographic information, symptoms, and laboratory results. By combining the results of many decision trees, random forest models improve prediction accuracy and stability, while reducing the risk of overfitting that can occur with a single decision tree. Each tree in the forest considers a random subset of features at each split, encouraging diverse model structures and robust performance. Although the overall model is less visually transparent than a single tree, random forests can provide valuable insights through measures of variable importance, helping clinicians and researchers understand which predictors most influence patient classification or risk assessment. This makes random forest a powerful and flexible tool for evidence-based decision-making and population health management.

Each decision tree within the random forest is built using recursive splits based on impurity measures such as Gini impurity or information gain (entropy), as mentioned above for the decision tree model. More formally, if there are M trees and $h_m(x)$ is the predicted class from tree m_i,then the final prediction is:

$$\widehat{y} = \text{majority\_vote}\ (h_1(x), h_2(x), \ldots, h_M(x))$$

In other words, random forest models leverage the recursive splitting criteria of decision trees (using Gini impurity or information gain) but aggregate the outputs of many such trees to improve predictive performance and stability. There is no single formula for the overall model; rather, the ensemble voting or averaging mechanism defines the final prediction process.

Titanic Data Example

We continue to use the Titanic dataset for this demonstration, predicting survival based on the same set of variables. Additionally, we utilize ChatGPT to generate clear, step-by-step R code by using a prompt such as: "Provide R code to apply a random forest model on the Titanic dataset, including model fitting, visualization, and interpretation of output." The code shown in Fig. 4.9 assumes that the data preparation steps used for the decision tree model have already been performed, allowing the same transformed variables to be reused:

The R code generated by ChatGPT demonstrates how to apply the random forest classification algorithm using the Titanic dataset. This process involves loading the

r Copy Edit

```r
# Load package
library(randomForest)
library(caret) # for confusionMatrix

# Fit Random Forest model
rf_model <- randomForest(
  Survived ~ Pclass + Sex + Age,
  data = train_data,      # assumes train_data already prepared
  ntree = 500,
  mtry = 2,
  importance = TRUE
)

# Predict on test data
rf_preds <- predict(rf_model, newdata = test_data, type = "class")

# Confusion matrix
confusionMatrix(rf_preds, test_data$Survived)
```

Fig. 4.9 R code generated by ChatGPT regarding how the random forest algorithm is performed in RStudio

necessary libraries, preparing the variables (such as Survived, Pclass, Sex, and Age), splitting the data into training and testing sets, fitting the random forest model, and evaluating its performance using predictions and a confusion matrix. These steps help ensure that the analysis is clear, reproducible, and useful for public health professionals interested in accurate risk prediction for outcomes like survival.

Similar to other models, we ask ChatGPT to explain what each part of the code does by prompting: "Provide explanations about what the random forest code was doing in RStudio." As expected, ChatGPT would then return clear, step-by-step interpretations for each line of code to support learning and application (see Fig. 4.10).

Evaluating Classification Models

After training a classification model, it is essential to assess how well it performs in predicting outcomes for new, unseen data. Effective evaluation not only quantifies the model's accuracy but also reveals strengths and weaknesses in identifying different outcome categories, which is crucial for public health and management decision-making (Hastie et al., 2009).

1) Load required packages

r Copy Edit

```r
library(randomForest)
library(caret)
```

- `randomForest` : contains the `randomForest()` function to fit the ensemble model.
- `caret` : provides the `confusionMatrix()` function to evaluate classification performance.

2) Fit the Random Forest model

r Copy Edit

```r
rf_model <- randomForest(
  Survived ~ Pclass + Sex + Age,
  data = train_data,
  ntree = 500,
  mtry = 2,
  importance = TRUE
)
```

- `Survived ~ Pclass + Sex + Age` : Formula — predicts `Survived` using `Pclass` , `Sex` , and `Age` .
- `data = train_data` : Uses the training dataset prepared earlier (already cleaned and with factors set).
- `ntree = 500` : Builds 500 decision trees in the ensemble.
- `mtry = 2` : At each split, the algorithm randomly considers 2 predictors out of the total available.
- `importance = TRUE` : Stores variable importance measures, which can later be plotted with `varImpPlot()` .

3) Make predictions on the test set

r Copy Edit

```r
rf_preds <- predict(rf_model, newdata = test_data, type = "class")
```

- Uses the fitted Random Forest model to predict the survival class for passengers in `test_data` .
- `type = "class"` returns the predicted class labels (not probabilities).

4) Evaluate model performance

r Copy Edit

```r
confusionMatrix(rf_preds, test_data$Survived)
```

- Compares predicted classes (`rf_preds`) with actual survival outcomes in the test data.
- Outputs:
  - **Accuracy**: Overall proportion of correct predictions.
  - **Sensitivity**: Proportion of actual survivors correctly predicted.
  - **Specificity**: Proportion of actual non-survivors correctly predicted.
  - Other metrics like Kappa for agreement.

Fig. 4.10 Explanations generated by ChatGPT regarding how the random forest algorithm is performed in RStudio

The Confusion (Contingency) Matrix

A fundamental tool for evaluating classification models is the *confusion matrix*, also known as the *contingency matrix*. Table 4.1 compares the model's predictions with the actual observed outcomes in the test dataset. For a binary classification problem, the matrix includes four key values (Fawcett, 2006):

In the confusion matrix shown as Table 4.1, the rows indicate "actual," whereas the columns indicate "predicted." That is, the first row is the number of observations with an actual value of "Yes" or commonly coded as "1." The second row is the number of observations with an actual value of "No" or commonly coded as "0." Each row is divided by whether the predicted value is "Yes" or "No," resulting in four possible cells:

- *True Positive (TP):* Model correctly predicts the positive class (e.g., disease present).
- *True Negative (TN):* Model correctly predicts the negative class (e.g., disease absent).
- *False Positive (FP):* Model incorrectly predicts positive when the actual is negative.
- *False Negative (FN):* Model incorrectly predicts negative when the actual is positive.

For example, an ML model is built to predict if patients have a substance use disorder (SUD). While the dataset already had the value of whether SUD is present, the researcher was interested in utilizing the dataset to build an ML model to predict the presence of SUD for future patients. Suppose the dataset had 100 patients. 50 of them actually had SUD, and 50 of them actually did not have SUD. Among the 50 "actual yes" patients, the model correctly predicted 20 of them had SUD (labeled as "True Positive" in Table 4.1), and incorrectly predicted 30 of them had no SUD ("False Negative"). Similarly, among the 50 "actual no" patients, the model incorrectly predicted 40 of them had SUD ("False Positive"), and correctly predicted 10 of them had no SUD ("True Negative"). Table 4.2 illustrates the distribution:

From this matrix, several key performance metrics can be calculated:

- *Accuracy:* Proportion of correct predictions, i.e., (TP + TN) / (TP + FN + FP + TN). In Table 4.2, it is (20 + 10)/(25 + 25 + 25 + 25) = 30/100 or 0.3.
- *Sensitivity (also known as Recall):* Ability to correctly identify positives, i.e., TP/(TP + FN). In Table 4.2, it is 20/(20 + 30) = 20/50 or 0.4.
- *Specificity:* Ability to correctly identify negatives, i.e., TN/(FP + TN). In Table 4.2, it is 10/(40 + 10) = 10/50 or 0.2.

Table 4.1 Confusion contingency matrix (also known as contingency matrix)

	Predicted: Yes (or "1")	Predicted: No (or "0")
Actual: Yes (or "1")	True Positive	False Negative
Actual: No (or "0")	False Positive	True Negative

Table 4.2 Confusion matrix of 100 imaginary patients

	Predicted: SUD (or "1")	Predicted: No SUD (or "0")
Actual: SUD (or "1")	20 (True Positive or TP)	30 (False Negative or FN)
Actual: No SUD (or "0")	40 (False Positive or FP)	10 (True Negative or TN)

- *Precision:* Proportion of predicted positives that are actually positive, i.e., TP / (TP + FP). In Table 4.2, it is 20/(20 + 40) = 20/60 or 0.33.

These metrics provide a more comprehensive understanding of the model's performance than accuracy alone, especially when the classes are imbalanced. Later chapters will utilize these metrics to illustrate how ML models may be evaluated and compared.

Comparison of Classification Models

A variety of supervised learning models are available for classification tasks in public health and management studies. While these models share a common goal—to predict categorical outcomes from observed features—they differ in methodology, interpretability, and specific application. Table 4.3 summarizes their key similarities and differences, as well as the datasets used and their primary purposes:

All four models share important similarities: they require splitting data into training and test sets, are designed for classification tasks, and can be implemented using R code as demonstrated in earlier sections. Despite these commonalities, the models differ in several respects, including their complexity, degree of interpretability, sensitivity to the scaling of input features, and the way predictions are generated.

Different datasets were used to illustrate each model in this chapter. The K-Nearest Neighbors (KNN) model was demonstrated using the iris dataset, which classifies flower species and is analogous to risk group classification in health contexts. Logistic regression was illustrated with the mtcars dataset, which predicts binary transmission type and serves as a parallel to binary health outcome prediction. Both the decision tree and random forest models were applied to the Titanic dataset, where the goal is to predict survival, similar to modeling health event outcomes.

When selecting among these models, it is important to consider their unique strengths. KNN is most intuitive for small, well-scaled datasets where the interpretability of distance-based similarity is valuable. Logistic regression is often preferred for its transparency and straightforward interpretation, particularly when the relationship between predictors and outcome is expected to be approximately linear. Decision tree models are highly interpretable and are especially useful for revealing important cutoff values and interactions among predictors. Random forest is best suited for more complex datasets with many variables and potential non-linear relationships, particularly when maximizing prediction accuracy is more important than interpretability.

Table 4.3 Comparison of 4 supervised learning models for classification: KNN, logistic regression, decision tree, and random forest

Model	Key features	Purpose/ Typical use	Illustrative dataset	Similarities	Differences
K-Nearest Neighbors (KNN)	Instance-based, non-parametric; predicts based on “closest” neighbors	Classifying new cases based on similarity to known cases	iris	Requires training/testing split; classification task	No model coefficients; sensitive to data scaling; parameter k must be chosen
Logistic regression	Parametric, interpretable; predicts probability of binary outcome	Predicting risk (e.g., disease presence/ absence)	mtcars	Requires training/testing split; classification task	Outputs probabilities and odds ratios; assumes linear relationship between predictors and log-odds
Decision tree	Rule-based, tree structure; interpretable flowchart of decisions	Identifying key predictors and decision thresholds	Titanic	Requires training/testing split; classification task	Handles both categorical and continuous features; visual, easy to interpret
Random Forest	Ensemble of decision trees; aggregates multiple tree predictions	Complex risk prediction; handles many predictors	Titanic	Requires training/testing split; classification task	Reduces overfitting; less interpretable than a single tree; provides variable importance measures

Together, these four models provide foundational approaches for supervised classification and can be adapted to address a wide range of public health problems.

Discussion Questions

1. What are the strengths and limitations of commonly used classification models (e.g., logistic regression, decision trees, KNN) in public health or management applications?
2. How does the choice of evaluation metrics (e.g., accuracy, precision, recall, F1 score, AUC) affect how we interpret the performance of a classification model?
3. When working with imbalanced datasets—such as rare disease detection—what strategies can be used to improve model performance and fairness?
4. How does model interpretability influence decision-making in high-stakes environments like healthcare or public policy?
5. What are the potential consequences of overfitting or underfitting a classification model, and how can these be detected and mitigated?

References

Breiman, L. (2001). Random forests. *Machine Learning, 45*(1), 5–32.
Breiman, L., Friedman, J., Stone, C. J., & Olshen, R. A. (1984). *Classification and regression trees*. CRC Press.
Esteva, A., Kuprel, B., Novoa, R. A., Ko, J., Swetter, S. M., Blau, H. M., & Thrun, S. (2017). Dermatologist-level classification of skin cancer with deep neural networks. *Nature, 542*(7639), 115–118. https://pubmed.ncbi.nlm.nih.gov/28117445/
Esteva, A., Robicquet, A., Ramsundar, B., Kuleshov, V., DePristo, M., Chou, K., Cui, C., Corrado, G., Thrun, S., & Dean, J. (2019). A guide to deep learning in healthcare. *Nature Medicine, 25*(1), 24–29. https://doi.org/10.1038/s41591-018-0316-z
Fawcett, T. (2006). An introduction to ROC analysis. *Pattern Recognition Letters, 27*(8), 861–874. https://doi.org/10.1016/j.patrec.2005.10.010
Goodfellow, I., Bengio, Y., & Courville, A. (2016). *Deep learning*. MIT Press. https://www.deeplearningbook.org/
Hastie, T., Tibshirani, R., & Friedman, J. (2009). *The elements of statistical learning: Data mining, inference, and prediction* (2nd ed.). Springer.
Hosmer, D. W., Lemeshow, S., & Sturdivant, R. X. (2013). *Applied logistic regression* (3rd ed.). Wiley.
Leung, R. C., Li, J., & Erdmann, C. (2017). Hospital readmission after post-acute care: Analyzing data from electronic health records. *Academy of Management Proceedings, 2016*(1), 11083. https://doi.org/10.5465/ambpp.2016.11083abstract
Rajkomar, A., Dean, J., & Kohane, I. (2019). Machine learning in medicine. *New England Journal of Medicine, 380*(14), 1347–1358. https://doi.org/10.1056/NEJMra1814259
Samuel, A. L. (1959). Some studies in machine learning using the game of checkers. *IBM Journal of Research and Development, 3*(3), 210–229. https://dl.acm.org/doi/10.1147/rd.33.0210
Xie, Z., Nikolayeva, O., Luo, J., & Li, D. (2019). Building risk prediction models for type 2 diabetes using machine learning techniques. *Preventing Chronic Disease, 16*, 190109. https://doi.org/10.5888/pcd16.190109

Chapter 5
Supervised Learning II: Regression Models

Learning Objectives

By the end of this chapter, students will be able to:

1. **Explain** the differences among major regression models in machine learning.
2. **Apply** regression models to real-world datasets.
3. **Evaluate** and **interpret** regression models using appropriate metrics.
4. **Use** R and RStudio to fit, assess, and visualize regression models.
5. **Leverage** AI tools like ChatGPT to generate R code and assist with troubleshooting and interpretation in regression modeling.

Introduction

In the previous chapter, we explored how machine learning (ML) enables computers to classify observations into discrete categories, such as disease presence or risk groups, by learning from labeled data. In this chapter, we extend these concepts to regression analysis in machine learning, which focuses on predicting continuous numerical outcomes rather than categorical labels.

Regression models in ML are used extensively in public health and management research to estimate values such as length of hospital stay, total healthcare costs, or laboratory measurements, given a set of predictor variables (James et al., 2013). For example, ML-based regression can predict a patient's expected length of stay based on their demographic and clinical characteristics, helping hospitals plan for staffing and resource allocation (Rajkomar et al., 2018). Similarly, regression models can forecast the costs associated with different treatment pathways or estimate future trends in key health indicators using large electronic health record (EHR) datasets

Supplementary Information The online version contains supplementary material available at https://doi.org/10.1007/978-3-032-08677-8_5.

R. Leung, *Leveraging GenAI for Machine Learning Education in Public Health*,
https://doi.org/10.1007/978-3-032-08677-8_5

(Obermeyer & Emanuel, 2016). These predictive capabilities provide critical, data-driven support for healthcare professionals and decision-makers.

As discussed in the previous chapter, a central feature of machine learning is how the data are handled during model development. Instead of using all available data at once—as is common in traditional statistical analyses—ML "recycles" the dataset by splitting it into distinct training and testing subsets (Hastie et al., 2009). The training data are used to build and calibrate the model, while the test data provide an objective measure of predictive accuracy on unseen cases. In some workflows, a third subset, known as a validation set, is used to fine-tune model parameters before final testing (Kuhn & Johnson, 2013). This approach is designed to ensure that ML regression models generalize well to new data, avoiding overfitting and enabling more robust, real-world prediction.

Throughout this chapter, we will introduce and compare four major regression models in machine learning, demonstrate their application using R and built-in datasets, and discuss best practices for evaluating and interpreting regression results. This structured approach mirrors the classification modeling process, reinforcing the common foundations and methodological rigor of supervised machine learning.

Supervised Learning for Regression Analysis

As discussed in the previous chapter, supervised learning is a foundational approach in machine learning that uses labeled data to train models for predicting new outcomes. In this chapter, we focus specifically on regression analysis, where the goal is to predict continuous numerical values rather than categorical labels.

Regression models are widely used in public health and management to estimate outcomes such as blood pressure, healthcare costs, hospital length of stay, or lab results (Chen & Asch, 2017). These models provide precise quantitative predictions that support effective decision-making and resource planning.

In the sections that follow, we will introduce four major regression models in machine learning:

1. **Linear Regression.**
2. **Polynomial Regression.**
3. **Ridge Regression.**
4. **Random Forest Regression.**

As in the previous chapter, we will also demonstrate how to utilize ChatGPT to assist with generating R code and understanding R scripts for each regression model. This approach will help you learn not only how to implement these models efficiently, but also how to interpret and troubleshoot your analysis in a practical and accessible way.

Training and Test Data in Regression Analysis

As introduced previously, dividing the dataset into training and test sets is a key principle in supervised machine learning, including regression analysis. This practice is crucial for developing regression models that make reliable, generalizable predictions and for ensuring that the evaluation of model performance accurately reflects real-world utility rather than how well the model "remembers" the training data (Friedman et al., 2001).

Why Use Training and Test Data?

- **Training data** is used to fit the regression model by showing the algorithm examples where both the predictor variables (such as age, weight, or lab results) and the actual numerical outcome (such as blood pressure, cost, or length of stay) are known. The model uses this data to learn the underlying relationships.
- **Test data** is held out and not used in the training process. It serves as an independent dataset for objectively assessing how well the model predicts outcomes for new, unseen observations. This helps identify overfitting, where a model appears accurate on training data but performs poorly on genuinely new data.

Importance in Regression Models

For regression analysis—where the goal is to predict continuous values rather than categories—splitting data ensures that model evaluation metrics such as **mean squared error (MSE)**, **root mean squared error (RMSE)**, and **R-squared** are unbiased. This approach is essential for validating the model's ability to generalize its predictions beyond the original data and is a standard practice across all major regression techniques.

Common Practice Across Regression Models

Splitting data into training and test sets is standard for all four regression models covered in this chapter: **linear regression**, **polynomial regression**, **ridge regression**, and **random forest regression**. Regardless of model complexity or mathematical approach, all require an unbiased evaluation using unseen data to ensure fair model comparison and trustworthy results in practical applications.

R Code for Data Splitting

The process of splitting data for regression analysis is essentially the same as in classification analysis. Using the caret package and its createDataPartition() function, the typical workflow is depicted in Fig. 5.1:

Linear Regression

Linear regression is a foundational and widely used machine learning algorithm for regression analysis, particularly suited for predicting continuous outcomes in public health and management. The goal of linear regression is to model the relationship between one or more predictor variables (features) and a continuous target variable by fitting a straight line through the observed data. This line represents the best linear approximation of the outcome as a function of the predictors, making it useful for quantifying trends, estimating effects, and forecasting future values.

The linear regression model predicts outcomes using the following equation:

$$\hat{y} = \beta_0 + \beta_1 x_1 + \beta_2 x_2 + \ldots + \beta_p x_p$$

r Copy Edit

```r
# Load caret
library(caret)

# Example: Use built-in mtcars dataset
data(mtcars)

# Set seed for reproducibility
set.seed(123)

# Create training (70%) and testing (30%) index
trainIndex <- createDataPartition(mtcars$mpg, p = 0.7, list = FALSE)

# Split the data
train_data <- mtcars[trainIndex, ]
test_data  <- mtcars[-trainIndex, ]
```

Fig. 5.1 Data partition steps generated by ChatGPT using the mtcars dataset

where:

- $\widehat{y}$ is the predicted outcome,
- β_0 is the intercept,
- $\beta_1, \beta_2, \ldots \beta_n$ are the coefficients for each predictor (also called "feature" in ML),
- $x_1, x_2, \ldots x_p$ are the predictor (also called "feature" in ML).

The coefficients are determined by minimizing the sum of squared residuals—the squared differences between observed and predicted values—using a method known as ordinary least squares (OLS).

Mtcars Dataset Example

To clearly illustrate linear regression, we use the built-in R dataset mtcars. This dataset includes various automobile attributes, such as miles per gallon (mpg), weight (wt), horsepower (hp), and number of cylinders (cyl). Here, we demonstrate how to predict mpg (fuel efficiency) using weight, horsepower, and cylinders as predictor variables.

ChatGPT can simplify the process of implementing linear regression in R by providing clear, step-by-step code. For example, a user might prompt: "Provide R code to apply linear regression on the mtcars dataset, including model fitting, interpretation, and evaluation."

The R code generated by ChatGPT demonstrates the process of applying linear regression using the mtcars dataset (see Fig. 5.2). It follows a structured workflow: loading the necessary libraries, importing and splitting the dataset into training and testing subsets, fitting the linear regression model to the training data, making predictions on the test data, and evaluating model performance using standard metrics such as mean squared error (MSE), root mean squared error (RMSE), and R-squared. This workflow enhances clarity, reproducibility, and interpretability, making it especially valuable for public health professionals developing regression models for predicting continuous clinical or management outcomes.

To better understand the specific actions performed by the above R code, we can enter a prompt such as "provide explanations about what the codes were doing in RStudio." The following detailed explanations would be returned (see Fig. 5.3):

Following the mtcars example above, linear regression can be directly applied to Electronic Health Records (EHR) to predict hospital length of stay—measured as the number of days a patient remains hospitalized—based on a set of clinical and demographic variables. In this scenario, linear regression uses features such as patient age, body mass index (BMI), severity of illness, comorbidities, and initial lab results to estimate the expected length of hospitalization for each new patient.

Within a machine learning context, linear regression operates according to the same mathematical foundations as traditional statistics but is embedded in a more predictive and validation-focused workflow (Bishop, 2006). Unlike traditional linear regression, which typically analyzes all available data at once and emphasizes

```r
# Linear regression on mtcars: fit, interpret, evaluate
library(caret)

# Load the data
data(mtcars)

# Set random seed for reproducibility
set.seed(123)

# Split data: 80% training, 20% testing
trainIndex <- createDataPartition(mtcars$mpg, p = 0.8, list = FALSE)
train_data <- mtcars[trainIndex, ]
test_data  <- mtcars[-trainIndex, ]

# Fit linear regression model on training data
lm_model <- lm(mpg ~ wt + hp + cyl, data = train_data)

# View summary of the model
summary(lm_model)

# Predictions on the test set
pred_mpg <- predict(lm_model, newdata = test_data)

# Evaluate model performance
mse <- mean((test_data$mpg - pred_mpg)^2)
rmse <- sqrt(mse)

# Calculate R-squared in two steps for readability
ss_res <- sum((test_data$mpg - pred_mpg)^2)
ss_tot <- sum((test_data$mpg - mean(test_data$mpg))^2)
rsq <- 1 - ss_res / ss_tot

# Print evaluation metrics
print(paste("Test MSE:", round(mse, 2)))
print(paste("Test RMSE:", round(rmse, 2)))
print(paste("Test R-squared:", round(rsq, 2)))
```

Fig. 5.2 R code generated by ChatGPT to perform the linear regression algorithm on the mtcars dataset

inference (such as hypothesis testing and the interpretation of coefficients), ML linear regression prioritizes predictive accuracy and model generalizability. In practice, this means the available data are divided into training and test sets: the model is built on the training data and evaluated on the test set to assess how well it predicts hospital length of stay for patients not seen during model development. This helps detect overfitting and provides a more realistic measure of model performance in real-world applications.

1) Load caret

```r
library(caret)
```

- Loads the **caret** package, which provides tools for splitting data, building models, and evaluating them.

2) Load the data

```r
data(mtcars)
```

- Loads the built-in **mtcars** dataset into your R session.
- We'll predict `mpg` (miles per gallon) using other variables.

3) Set random seed

```r
set.seed(123)
```

- Ensures that the random data split is reproducible—important for consistent results if the code is run again.

Fig. 5.3 Explanations generated by ChatGPT to explain how the linear regression algorithm is performed in RStudio

By applying linear regression to large-scale EHR data using rigorous data partitioning, public health and hospital management professionals can make robust, data-driven forecasts about length of stay for individual patients. These predictions inform resource allocation, discharge planning, and operational efficiency in healthcare settings. This predictive and practical emphasis distinguishes machine learning-based linear regression from traditional approaches and highlights its value for modern healthcare analytics and decision support.

Polynomial Regression

Polynomial regression is an extension of linear regression that allows the model to capture non-linear relationships between predictor variables and a continuous outcome. While linear regression fits a straight line to the data, polynomial regression

9) Calculate R-squared for the test data

r Copy Edit

```r
ss_res <- sum((test_data$mpg - pred_mpg)^2)
ss_tot <- sum((test_data$mpg - mean(test_data$mpg))^2)
rsq <- 1 - ss_res / ss_tot
```

- **ss_res**: residual sum of squares (unexplained variation).
- **ss_tot**: total sum of squares (total variation in the data).
- **R²**: proportion of variance explained by the model on unseen data.

10) Print the evaluation metrics

r Copy Edit

```r
print(paste("Test MSE:", round(mse, 2)))
print(paste("Test RMSE:", round(rmse, 2)))
print(paste("Test R-squared:", round(rsq, 2)))
```

- Displays the MSE, RMSE, and R² values for quick performance assessment.
- Lower MSE/RMSE and higher R² indicate better model performance.

Fig. 5.3 (continued)

fits a curved line by including higher-order terms (such as squared or cubic predictors). This makes polynomial regression especially useful in public health and management when trends or effects are not strictly linear, such as modeling the rise and plateau of healthcare costs or physiological measurements over time.

The polynomial regression model predicts outcomes using the following equation:

$$\hat{y} = \beta_0 + \beta_1 x + \beta_2 x^2 + \beta_3 x^3 + \ldots + \beta_d x^d$$

where:

- $\hat{y}$ is the predicted outcome,
- β_0 is the intercept,
- $\beta_1, \beta_2, \ldots \beta_n$ are the coefficients for each predictor (also called "feature" in ML),
- x is the predictor (also called "feature" in ML) variable raised to increasing powers (2, 3, …, d).

As with linear regression, the coefficients are determined by minimizing the sum of squared residuals using ordinary least squares (OLS).

Mtcars Dataset Example

To illustrate polynomial regression, we again use the built-in R dataset mtcars. For this example, we predict miles per gallon (mpg) using car weight (wt), but we now allow for a non-linear relationship by including a squared term for weight. ChatGPT can help streamline the process of implementing polynomial regression in R. A user might prompt: "Provide R code to apply polynomial regression (including squared terms) on the mtcars dataset, including data splitting, model fitting, and evaluation."

Figure 5.4 presents an example of the R code that ChatGPT might generate:

r Copy Edit

```r
# 1) Load package
library(caret)

# 2) Load data
data(mtcars)

# 3) Reproducibility
set.seed(123)

# 4) Train/test split (80/20)
trainIndex <- createDataPartition(mtcars$mpg, p = 0.8, list = FALSE)
train_data <- mtcars[trainIndex, ]
test_data  <- mtcars[-trainIndex, ]

# 5) Fit polynomial regression with wt^2 (raw quadratic term)
poly_model <- lm(mpg ~ wt + I(wt^2), data = train_data)

# 6) Model summary
summary(poly_model)

# 7) Predictions on test set
pred_mpg <- predict(poly_model, newdata = test_data)

# 8) Evaluation metrics: MSE, RMSE, R-squared
mse  <- mean((test_data$mpg - pred_mpg)^2)
rmse <- sqrt(mse)
ss_res <- sum((test_data$mpg - pred_mpg)^2)
ss_tot <- sum((test_data$mpg - mean(test_data$mpg))^2)
rsq  <- 1 - ss_res / ss_tot

# 9) Print metrics
print(paste("Test MSE:", round(mse, 2)))
print(paste("Test RMSE:", round(rmse, 2)))
print(paste("Test R-squared:", round(rsq, 2)))
```

Fig. 5.4 R code generated by ChatGPT to perform the polynomial regression algorithm

This code demonstrates a standard workflow: loading libraries, splitting data, fitting the polynomial regression model to the training set, predicting on the test set, and evaluating performance using common metrics.

To better understand what each part of the code accomplishes, users can ask ChatGPT for detailed explanations of every step, from data preparation to model interpretation and diagnostics. We can enter a prompt such as "provide explanations about what the codes were doing in RStudio." The following detailed explanations would be returned (see Fig. 5.5):

1) Load package

r Copy Edit

```r
library(caret)
```

- Loads the **caret** package, which provides functions for splitting data and evaluating models.

2) Load data

r Copy Edit

```r
data(mtcars)
```

- Loads the built-in **mtcars** dataset.
- `mpg` (miles per gallon) will be the outcome, and `wt` (car weight) is the main predictor.

3) Reproducibility

r Copy Edit

```r
set.seed(123)
```

- Sets a fixed random seed so the train/test split is the same every time you run the code.

4) Train/test split (80/20)

r Copy Edit

```r
trainIndex <- createDataPartition(mtcars$mpg, p = 0.8, list = FALSE)
train_data <- mtcars[trainIndex, ]
test_data  <- mtcars[-trainIndex, ]
```

- `createDataPartition()` selects about 80% of the rows for training (`train_data`) and the rest for testing (`test_data`).
- Keeps the distribution of `mpg` similar in both sets.

Fig. 5.5 Explanations generated by ChatGPT regarding how the polynomial regression algorithm is performed in RStudio

5) Fit polynomial regression with wt^2

r Copy Edit

```
poly_model <- lm(mpg ~ wt + I(wt^2), data = train_data)
```

- Fits a **quadratic regression model**:

$$\text{mpg} = \beta_0 + \beta_1 \cdot \text{wt} + \beta_2 \cdot \text{wt}^2 + \epsilon$$

- `I(wt^2)` tells R to use the square of `wt` as a raw term, not as part of a formula operation.

6) Model summary

r Copy Edit

```
summary(poly_model)
```

- Displays estimated coefficients, statistical significance, and model fit metrics (R^2, Adjusted R^2) for the training set.
- Coefficient signs and magnitudes indicate the shape of the curve relating weight to mpg.

7) Predictions on the test set

r Copy Edit

```
pred_mpg <- predict(poly_model, newdata = test_data)
```

- Uses the fitted model to predict `mpg` for cars in the test set.

8) Evaluation metrics

r Copy Edit

```
mse  <- mean((test_data$mpg - pred_mpg)^2)
rmse <- sqrt(mse)
ss_res <- sum((test_data$mpg - pred_mpg)^2)
ss_tot <- sum((test_data$mpg - mean(test_data$mpg))^2)
rsq  <- 1 - ss_res / ss_tot
```

- **MSE**: average squared prediction error.
- **RMSE**: square root of MSE, in mpg units—easier to interpret.
- **R^2**: proportion of variance in mpg explained by the model on unseen data.

9) Print metrics

r Copy Edit

```
print(paste("Test MSE:", round(mse, 2)))
print(paste("Test RMSE:", round(rmse, 2)))
print(paste("Test R-squared:", round(rsq, 2)))
```

- Displays the three key performance metrics for quick interpretation.
- Lower MSE/RMSE and higher R^2 generally indicate better predictive performance.

Fig. 5.5 (continued)

Following the mtcars example above, polynomial regression can also be applied to Electronic Health Records (EHR) to predict hospital length of stay (measured in days) based on clinical and demographic features. In many cases, the relationship between a predictor (such as age or severity of illness) and length of stay is not simply linear—a curved or more complex relationship may exist. Polynomial regression accounts for this by including squared or higher-order terms of predictors, allowing the model to capture such non-linear effects.

Applying polynomial regression to large EHR datasets in this way enables health professionals and managers to generate more accurate forecasts for patient length of stay—especially when effects are not purely linear. This supports more informed decisions for resource allocation, discharge planning, and hospital operations, highlighting the practical value of ML-based polynomial regression in real-world healthcare management.

Ridge Regression

Ridge regression is an extension of linear regression designed to address challenges that arise when predictor variables are highly correlated (multicollinearity) or when there are a large number of predictors. While ordinary linear regression can produce unstable or overly large coefficients in such situations, ridge regression introduces a penalty term that "shrinks" the size of the coefficients, improving the model's generalizability and predictive accuracy (Hoerl & Kennard, 1970). This makes ridge regression especially valuable in public health and management studies where datasets may contain many interrelated features.

The ridge regression model estimates coefficients by minimizing a modified loss function:

$$\text{Minimize}: \sum_{i=1}^{n} (y_i - \widehat{y}_i)^2 + \lambda \sum_{j=1}^{p} \beta_j^2$$

where:

- y_i is the observed outcome for the i-th observation,
- $\widehat{y}_i$ is the predicted outcome,
- β_j are the model coefficients
- λ is the regularization (penalty) parameter controlling the amount of shrinkage,
- n is the number of observations,
- p is the number of predictors.

The penalty term $\lambda \sum_{j=1}^{p} \beta_j^2$ helps reduce overfitting by discouraging large coefficients.

Mtcars Dataset Example

To illustrate ridge regression, we use the built-in R dataset mtcars again. In this example, we predict miles per gallon (mpg) using weight (wt), horsepower (hp), and number of cylinders (cyl), applying ridge regression to handle potential multicollinearity among predictors. ChatGPT can help generate the required R code. For example, a user might prompt: "Provide R code to apply ridge regression on the mtcars dataset, including data splitting, model fitting with the glmnet package, and evaluation."

This code demonstrates how to load libraries, split the data, prepare variables for glmnet, fit the ridge regression model, make predictions, and evaluate performance using standard regression metrics (see Fig. 5.6). Users can also prompt ChatGPT to provide step-by-step explanations of each code section for a deeper understanding of the workflow and its purpose.

As with other ML models, users can prompt ChatGPT with queries like: "Provide step-by-step explanations about what the codes are doing in RStudio." ChatGPT would then generate detailed explanations clarifying each step in the workflow, as illustrated in Fig. 5.7:

Applying Ridge Regression to Health Data

Ridge regression is particularly valuable in health analytics when predicting continuous outcomes like hospital length of stay or treatment costs using many correlated features, such as multiple lab results or demographic factors. By penalizing overly complex models and shrinking coefficients, ridge regression supports more stable, generalizable predictions that are less sensitive to the quirks of any single dataset.

As with other ML regression models, data partitioning and independent test set evaluation are essential for assessing real-world predictive performance and guiding robust decision-making in healthcare and management.

Lasso Regression

Lasso regression is another variant of regularized regression, closely related to ridge regression, designed to address challenges of multicollinearity and high-dimensional datasets. Unlike ridge regression, which shrinks coefficient estimates toward zero, lasso regression can set coefficients exactly to zero, effectively performing feature selection (Tibshirani, 1996). This property makes lasso regression especially useful in public health and management studies, where datasets often contain many predictors, only some of which significantly contribute to predicting outcomes.

The lasso regression model estimates coefficients by minimizing the following modified loss function:

Example R code:

r Copy Edit

```r
# Load required libraries
library(caret)
library(glmnet)

# Load the dataset
data(mtcars)

# Set random seed for reproducibility
set.seed(123)

# Split data: 80% training, 20% testing
trainIndex <- createDataPartition(mtcars$mpg, p = 0.8, list = FALSE)
train_data <- mtcars[trainIndex, ]
test_data <- mtcars[-trainIndex, ]

# Prepare predictor matrix and response vector
x_train <- as.matrix(train_data[, c('wt', 'hp', 'cyl')])
y_train <- train_data$mpg
x_test <- as.matrix(test_data[, c('wt', 'hp', 'cyl')])
y_test <- test_data$mpg

# Fit ridge regression model (alpha = 0)
ridge_model <- glmnet(x_train, y_train, alpha = 0)

# Predict using the fitted model (selecting a reasonable lambda)
pred_mpg <- predict(ridge_model, s = 0.1, newx = x_test)

# Evaluate model performance
mse <- mean((y_test - pred_mpg)^2)
rmse <- sqrt(mse)
rsq <- 1 - sum((y_test - pred_mpg)^2) / sum((y_test - mean(y_test))^2)

print(paste("Test MSE:", round(mse, 2)))
print(paste("Test RMSE:", round(rmse, 2)))
print(paste("Test R-squared:", round(rsq, 2)))
```

This code walks through the workflow of loading libraries, splitting data, preparing matrices for `glmnet`, fitting the ridge regression model, making predictions, and evaluating test performance.

If users want further clarity, they can prompt ChatGPT with "provide explanations about what the codes were doing in R studio," and receive a step-by-step breakdown.

Fig. 5.6 R code generated by ChatGPT to perform the ridge regression algorithm

Step-by-Step Explanation of Ridge Regression Code in RStudio

Step 1: Load required libraries

r Copy Edit

```r
library(caret)
library(glmnet)
```

- `caret` provides convenient tools for data splitting, model training, and evaluation.
- `glmnet` allows fitting ridge (and other regularized) regression models.

Step 2: Load the dataset

r Copy Edit

```r
data(mtcars)
```

- Loads the built-in dataset `mtcars`, containing various automobile characteristics.

Step 3: Set random seed for reproducibility

r Copy Edit

```r
set.seed(123)
```

- Ensures consistent and reproducible results by controlling randomness in data splitting and modeling processes.

Step 4: Split data into training (80%) and testing (20%) sets

r Copy Edit

```r
trainIndex <- createDataPartition(mtcars$mpg, p = 0.8, list = FALSE)
train_data <- mtcars[trainIndex, ]
test_data <- mtcars[-trainIndex, ]
```

- Divides data into training and test subsets to allow unbiased evaluation of the model's predictive accuracy on unseen data.

Fig. 5.7 Explanations generated by ChatGPT regarding how the ridge regression algorithm is performed in RStudio

Step 5: Prepare predictor matrices and response vectors

r Copy Edit

```
x_train <- as.matrix(train_data[, c('wt', 'hp', 'cyl')])
y_train <- train_data$mpg
x_test <- as.matrix(test_data[, c('wt', 'hp', 'cyl')])
y_test <- test_data$mpg
```

- Converts predictor variables (`wt` , `hp` , `cyl`) into matrix format, which is required by the `glmnet` function.
- Separates the response variable (`mpg`) into vectors for training (`y_train`) and testing (`y_test`).

Step 6: Fit the ridge regression model (alpha = 0)

r Copy Edit

```
ridge_model <- glmnet(x_train, y_train, alpha = 0)
```

- Fits a ridge regression model to the training data.
- The parameter `alpha = 0` specifically denotes ridge regression (which shrinks coefficients toward zero, but does not eliminate predictors entirely).

Step 7: Predict on test data using the fitted model

r Copy Edit

```
pred_mpg <- predict(ridge_model, s = 0.1, newx = x_test)
```

- Predicts miles per gallon (`mpg`) values for the test dataset.
- The regularization parameter (`lambda`) is set at 0.1 here as a demonstration, but typically selected via cross-validation.

Fig. 5.7 (continued)

$$\text{Minimize}: \sum_{i=1}^{n} (y_i - \widehat{y}_i)^2 + \lambda \sum_{j=1}^{p} |\beta_j|$$

where:

- y_i is the observed outcome for the i-th observation,
- $\widehat{y}_i$ is the predicted outcome,
- β_j are the model coefficients
- λ is the regularization (penalty) parameter controlling the penalty strength.

Increasing λ penalizes large coefficients more aggressively, often pushing irrelevant predictor coefficients exactly to zero and thus performing automatic feature selection.

Step 8: Evaluate model performance using test data

r Copy Edit

```
mse <- mean((y_test - pred_mpg)^2)
rmse <- sqrt(mse)
rsq <- 1 - sum((y_test - pred_mpg)^2) / sum((y_test - mean(y_test))^2)

print(paste("Test MSE:", round(mse, 2)))
print(paste("Test RMSE:", round(rmse, 2)))
print(paste("Test R-squared:", round(rsq, 2)))
```

- Calculates three standard metrics:
  - **Mean Squared Error (MSE)**: Average of squared differences between actual and predicted values.
  - **Root Mean Squared Error (RMSE)**: The square root of MSE, indicating prediction error magnitude.
  - **R-squared (R^2)**: Proportion of variance in the outcome explained by the model.
- The printed values indicate how effectively the ridge regression model predicts new observations.

Fig. 5.7 (continued)

Mtcars Dataset Example

To illustrate lasso regression, we again use the built-in R dataset mtcars. We predict miles per gallon (mpg) using several car features (wt, hp., and cyl), applying lasso regression to handle multicollinearity and perform automatic variable selection.

ChatGPT can assist in generating the required R code. A user might prompt: "Provide R code to apply lasso regression on the mtcars dataset, including data splitting, model fitting with the glmnet package, and evaluation" (see Fig. 5.8).

To further understand this code, a user could prompt ChatGPT: "Provide step-by-step explanations about what the codes are doing in RStudio." Detailed explanations would then clarify each step in the workflow (see Fig. 5.9).

Applying Lasso Regression to Health Data

Lasso regression is particularly valuable in health analytics when predicting continuous outcomes, such as hospital length of stay, readmission rates, or medical costs, using large datasets containing multiple correlated predictors. By performing automatic feature selection and penalizing overly complex models, lasso regression generates simpler, more interpretable, and often more accurate predictive models.

Here is the R code example that ChatGPT might provide:

r Copy Edit

```r
# Load required libraries
library(caret)
library(glmnet)

# Load dataset
data(mtcars)

# Set random seed for reproducibility
set.seed(123)

# Split data into training and testing sets (80%-20%)
trainIndex <- createDataPartition(mtcars$mpg, p = 0.8, list = FALSE)
train_data <- mtcars[trainIndex, ]
test_data <- mtcars[-trainIndex, ]

# Prepare predictor matrices and response vectors
x_train <- as.matrix(train_data[, c("wt", "hp", "cyl")])
y_train <- train_data$mpg
x_test <- as.matrix(test_data[, c("wt", "hp", "cyl")])
y_test <- test_data$mpg

# Fit lasso regression model (alpha = 1 for lasso)
lasso_model <- glmnet(x_train, y_train, alpha = 1)

# Select optimal lambda using cross-validation
cv_lasso <- cv.glmnet(x_train, y_train, alpha = 1)
best_lambda <- cv_lasso$lambda.min

# Make predictions on test data
pred_mpg <- predict(lasso_model, s = best_lambda, newx = x_test)

# Evaluate model performance
mse <- mean((y_test - pred_mpg)^2)
rmse <- sqrt(mse)

print(paste("Test MSE:", round(mse, 2)))
print(paste("Test RMSE:", round(rmse, 2)))
```

This code covers loading libraries, data splitting, preparing variables for `glmnet`, selecting the optimal lambda via cross-validation, fitting the lasso model, making predictions, and evaluating performance.

Fig. 5.8 R code generated by ChatGPT to perform the lasso regression algorithm

As with other ML regression methods, rigorous data partitioning and evaluation on independent test sets are essential to ensure real-world generalizability and to guide reliable, evidence-based decision-making in healthcare and management contexts.

Step-by-Step Explanation of Lasso Regression Code in RStudio

Step 1: Load required libraries

r Copy Edit

```r
library(caret)
library(glmnet)
```

- `caret` is used for convenient data partitioning and model evaluation.
- `glmnet` is specialized for fitting regularized regression models (ridge and lasso).

Step 2: Load the built-in dataset

r Copy Edit

```r
data(mtcars)
```

- Loads the `mtcars` dataset, containing automobile data.

Step 3: Set random seed for reproducibility

r Copy Edit

```r
set.seed(123)
```

- Ensures that the random processes (e.g., data splitting) are reproducible, producing the same results each time the code is run.

Step 4: Split the data into training and testing sets

r Copy Edit

```r
trainIndex <- createDataPartition(mtcars$mpg, p = 0.8, list = FALSE)
train_data <- mtcars[trainIndex, ]
test_data <- mtcars[-trainIndex, ]
```

- `createDataPartition` splits data, with 80% assigned to training and 20% to testing.
- `train_data` is used to fit the model, while `test_data` evaluates performance on unseen data.

Fig. 5.9 Explanations generated by ChatGPT regarding how the ridge regression algorithm is performed in RStudio

Step 5: Prepare predictor matrices and response vectors

r Copy Edit

```
x_train <- as.matrix(train_data[, c("wt", "hp", "cyl")])
y_train <- train_data$mpg
x_test <- as.matrix(test_data[, c("wt", "hp", "cyl")])
y_test <- test_data$mpg
```

- Converts predictor variables into matrices, which `glmnet` requires.
- Separates the outcome variable (`mpg`) into a distinct vector for training (`y_train`) and testing (`y_test`).

Step 6: Fit the initial lasso regression model

r Copy Edit

```
lasso_model <- glmnet(x_train, y_train, alpha = 1)
```

- Fits a lasso regression model using training data.
- The parameter `alpha = 1` specifically indicates lasso regression (setting some coefficients exactly to zero).

Step 7: Select the optimal penalty parameter (lambda) via cross-validation

r Copy Edit

```
cv_lasso <- cv.glmnet(x_train, y_train, alpha = 1)
best_lambda <- cv_lasso$lambda.min
```

- Performs cross-validation to identify the optimal value of lambda (penalty strength).
- `lambda.min` selects the value that provides the smallest prediction error.

Step 8: Predict outcomes on the test data using the optimal lambda

r Copy Edit

```
pred_mpg <- predict(lasso_model, s = best_lambda, newx = x_test)
```

- Generates predicted values (`pred_mpg`) for the test dataset using the selected optimal lambda.

Fig. 5.9 (continued)

Step 9: Evaluate model performance on the test set

r Copy Edit

```
mse <- mean((y_test - pred_mpg)^2)
rmse <- sqrt(mse)

print(paste("Test MSE:", round(mse, 2)))
print(paste("Test RMSE:", round(rmse, 2)))
```

- Calculates **Mean Squared Error (MSE)**, indicating the average squared difference between predicted and actual values.
- Calculates **Root Mean Squared Error (RMSE)**, a measure of prediction accuracy expressed in original units (`mpg`).
- Prints these metrics, summarizing how effectively the model generalizes to unseen data.

These steps collectively describe how lasso regression is practically implemented and evaluated within R, providing clarity on each aspect of the model-building process.

Fig. 5.9 (continued)

Evaluation of Regression Models

Evaluating regression models involves assessing how accurately the models predict continuous outcomes (Hastie et al., 2009). Key metrics include:

- *Mean Squared Error (MSE):* Measures the average squared difference between the observed and predicted values, emphasizing larger errors.
- *Root Mean Squared Error (RMSE):* The square root of MSE, expressed in the same units as the outcome, providing intuitive interpretation.
- *R-squared (R^2):* Represents the proportion of variance in the dependent variable explained by the model, indicating how well the model fits the data.

Using ChatGPT, a user can enter a prompt such as "show example codes in RStudio to evaluate ML regression models" to see examples of R scripts (that can be used in both R and RStudio) to evaluate ML regression models. The following results return (see Fig. 5.10):

Table 5.1 provides a comparison of the four regression models discussed in this chapter. It highlights key features, the ability to handle non-linearity, control for overfitting, interpretability, illustrative dataset(s), and typical applications.

Here is a concise and clear example of how you can evaluate machine learning regression models in RStudio:

r Copy Edit

```r
# Example codes to evaluate regression models in R

# Assuming actual_mpg are true observed values, pred_mpg are model predictions

# Mean Squared Error (MSE)
mse <- mean((actual_mpg - pred_mpg)^2)

# Root Mean Squared Error (RMSE)
rmse <- sqrt(mse)

# R-squared (R²)
rsq <- 1 - sum((actual_mpg - pred_mpg)^2) / sum((actual_mpg - mean(actual_mpg))^2)

# Display the evaluation metrics
print(paste("Mean Squared Error (MSE):", round(mse, 2)))
print(paste("Root Mean Squared Error (RMSE):", round(rmse, 2)))
print(paste("R-squared (R²):", round(rsq, 2)))
```

Explanation:

- **Mean Squared Error (MSE)** quantifies the average squared difference between the observed and predicted values.
- **Root Mean Squared Error (RMSE)** provides the error in the original outcome units, making it easier to interpret.
- **R-squared (R^2)** indicates the proportion of variance in the outcome that the model explains, measuring the model's goodness-of-fit.

Fig. 5.10 Explanations generated by ChatGPT regarding how ML regression models can be evaluated in RStudio

Regression Model Comparison Table

Table 5.1 Comparison of 4 supervised learning models for regression: linear regression, polynomial regression, ridge regression, and lasso regression

Model	Key features	Handles non-linearity	Controls overfitting	Interpretability	Illustrative dataset	Typical applications
Linear regression	Simple linear relationships	No	No	High	mtcars	Trend analysis, explanatory modeling
Polynomial regression	Incorporates polynomial terms	Yes	No	Moderate	mtcars	Non-linear trends, growth patterns
Ridge regression	Penalizes coefficients (L2 penalty)	No	Yes	Moderate	mtcars	Correlated predictors, feature stability
Lasso regression	Penalizes coefficients (L1 penalty)	No	Yes	High (feature selection)	mtcars	High-dimensional data, feature selection

Summary

This chapter introduced and compared four foundational regression models—linear, polynomial, ridge, and lasso—highlighting their practical applications using R's built-in datasets. Understanding these models and evaluation metrics empowers researchers and managers to select appropriate methods for accurate prediction and effective decision-making. Proper data preparation, rigorous evaluation, and clear interpretation remain critical for robust regression modeling in public health and management contexts.

Discussion Questions

1. What factors would you consider when choosing between linear regression, polynomial regression, ridge regression, and lasso regression in a healthcare context?
2. Why is it essential to split data into training and test sets in machine learning regression? Discuss potential consequences of not following this practice.
3. How would you explain the importance of evaluation metrics like Mean Squared Error (MSE), Root Mean Squared Error (RMSE), and R-squared (R^2) to a healthcare management team?
4. In what scenarios would you prefer ridge regression over lasso regression and vice versa? How does each model help manage overfitting and multicollinearity?
5. Discuss the benefits and possible limitations of using AI-driven tools such as ChatGPT to assist in the regression modeling process, specifically in terms of generating code and interpreting results.

References

Bishop, C. M. (2006). *Pattern recognition and machine learning*. Springer. https://www.springer.com/gp/book/9780387310732

Chen, J. H., & Asch, S. M. (2017). Machine learning and prediction in medicine—Beyond the peak of inflated expectations. *New England Journal of Medicine, 376*(26), 2507–2509. https://doi.org/10.1056/NEJMp1702071

Friedman, J., Hastie, T., & Tibshirani, R. (2001). *The elements of statistical learning: Data mining, inference, and prediction*. Springer. https://web.stanford.edu/~hastie/ElemStatLearn/

Hastie, T., Tibshirani, R., & Friedman, J. (2009). *The elements of statistical learning: Data mining, inference, and prediction* (2nd ed.). Springer. https://web.stanford.edu/~hastie/ElemStatLearn/

Hoerl, A. E., & Kennard, R. W. (1970). Ridge regression: Biased estimation for nonorthogonal problems. *Technometrics, 12*(1), 55–67. https://doi.org/10.1080/00401706.1970.10488634

James, G., Witten, D., Hastie, T., & Tibshirani, R. (2013). *An introduction to statistical learning: With applications in R*. Springer. https://www.statlearning.com/

Kuhn, M., & Johnson, K. (2013). *Applied predictive modeling*. Springer. https://doi.org/10.1007/978-1-4614-6849-3

Obermeyer, Z., & Emanuel, E. J. (2016). Predicting the future—Big data, machine learning, and clinical medicine. *New England Journal of Medicine, 375*(13), 1216–1219. https://doi.org/10.1056/NEJMp1606181

Rajkomar, A., Oren, E., Chen, K., Dai, A. M., Hajaj, N., Hardt, M., et al. (2018). Scalable and accurate deep learning with electronic health records. *npj Digital Medicine, 1*(1), 1–10. https://doi.org/10.1038/s41746-018-0029-1

Tibshirani, R. (1996). Regression shrinkage and selection via the lasso. *Journal of the Royal Statistical Society: Series B (Methodological), 58*(1), 267–288. https://doi.org/10.1111/j.2517-6161.1996.tb02080.x

Chapter 6
Unsupervised Learning

Learning Objectives
By the end of this chapter, students will be able to:

1. **Understand** the core principles of unsupervised learning and its value in management and health analytics.
2. **Apply** clustering and dimensionality reduction techniques in R.
3. **Interpret** results and visualize clusters or data structures.
4. **Use** AI tools like ChatGPT to generate and explain R code for unsupervised learning tasks.

Introduction

Machine learning (ML) empowers computers to detect meaningful patterns in data, making it invaluable for analyzing complex datasets where outcomes or labels may not be initially known. Unlike supervised learning—which relies on labeled data—unsupervised learning explores the inherent structure within unlabeled data (Hastie et al., 2009). This approach focuses on discovering natural organization and relationships within the data without predefined labels or outcomes (Bishop, 2006). It is widely used in public health and management studies for segmenting populations, identifying trends, and reducing data complexity (Jain, 2010).

In healthcare, unsupervised learning can cluster patient populations based on clinical characteristics, enabling tailored interventions and more precise resource allocation (Miotto et al., 2016). For example, unsupervised ML algorithms may uncover distinct groups of patients with similar health profiles or healthcare usage

Supplementary Information The online version contains supplementary material available at https://doi.org/10.1007/978-3-032-08677-8_6.

R. Leung, *Leveraging GenAI for Machine Learning Education in Public Health*,
https://doi.org/10.1007/978-3-032-08677-8_6

patterns (Tomar & Agarwal, 2013). These insights are critical for strategic planning, targeted preventive care, and personalized treatment pathways (Rajkomar et al., 2018).

A key advantage of unsupervised learning is that it requires no prior knowledge or outcome labels. Instead, the algorithms autonomously detect underlying patterns, groupings, or anomalies (MacQueen, 1967). Common techniques include clustering, dimensionality reduction, and anomaly detection. These methods enable exploratory data analysis and help researchers interpret complex, multidimensional healthcare datasets, ultimately supporting hypothesis generation and informed decision-making (Likas et al., 2003).

Unsupervised Learning Models

In this chapter, we will introduce three major models of unsupervised learning—K-means clustering, hierarchical clustering, and principal component analysis (PCA)—and demonstrate each using R's built-in datasets and practical code examples. As in previous chapters, we will also show how ChatGPT can assist with coding and interpretation, helping users implement and understand these techniques in RStudio efficiently.

K-Means Clustering K-means is a partition-based clustering algorithm that groups observations into a pre-specified number of clusters based on feature similarity (MacQueen, 1967). It is particularly useful for identifying patient segments, treatment profiles, or behavioral patterns from structured health data.

Hierarchical Clustering Hierarchical clustering creates a tree-like structure (dendrogram) that illustrates how individual elements or clusters are merged or split based on distance metrics (Johnson, 1967). This method is especially useful for subgroup discovery, classification hierarchies, and understanding nested relationships among data points.

Principal Component Analysis (PCA) PCA is a dimensionality reduction technique that transforms a large set of variables into a smaller one that still contains most of the information (Pearson, 1901; Hotelling, 1933). It simplifies visualization, improves model performance, and is valuable for detecting patterns in high-dimensional health datasets.

Training and Testing in Unsupervised Learning

Unlike supervised learning, unsupervised learning does not rely on outcome labels, so the concepts of training and testing data are less formally defined. However, evaluation is still important, particularly for assessing the stability and usefulness of discovered patterns or reduced dimensions (Hennig, 2007). In clustering, for example, techniques such as silhouette scores or cross-validation on subsamples of the data may be used to evaluate clustering quality (Rousseeuw, 1987). For dimensionality reduction methods like PCA, the proportion of variance explained by each component provides insight into how well the model captures the original data structure. While unsupervised models do not "learn" in the same way as supervised algorithms, it is still good practice to evaluate their robustness across different data splits or sampling conditions when applying them to real-world public health data.

K-Means Clustering

K-means clustering is a widely used unsupervised machine learning algorithm that partitions a dataset into a pre-specified number of clusters (k), with each observation assigned to the cluster with the nearest mean (centroid). In public health, K-means is especially useful for identifying population subgroups based on clinical, behavioral, or demographic variables—for example, segmenting patients by health risk, utilization patterns, or treatment response.

Unlike KNN, K-means does not rely on labeled training data. Instead, it groups observations by minimizing the within-cluster variance. The algorithm begins by randomly initializing k centroids and iteratively updates them by:

1. Assigning each observation to the nearest centroid (based on distance, typically Euclidean),
2. Recomputing the centroids as the mean of all observations in each cluster.

This process continues until cluster assignments no longer change or a maximum number of iterations is reached. Similar to KNN, K-means also relies on the Euclidean distance formula to measure similarity between observations:

$$d(x, y) = \sqrt{\sum_{i=1}^{n} (x_i - y_i)^2}$$

where:

- $d(x, y)$ is the Euclidean distance between observations x and y,
- x_i and y_i represent the respective values of feature i in the observations,
- n is the number of features.

Iris Dataset Example

To illustrate K-means clustering, we use the built-in R dataset iris. This dataset contains 150 samples from three iris species, each with four numeric variables (sepal length, sepal width, petal length, petal width). Although species labels are included, they are not used in K-means clustering, as the algorithm is unsupervised.

In ChatGPT, a user might prompt: "Provide R code to apply K-means clustering on the iris dataset, including visualization and evaluation." Based on this prompt, ChatGPT can generate R code that performs clustering, creates cluster plots, and compares cluster assignments to known species (for validation purposes only). This allows users to explore how well the algorithm uncovers natural groupings and to assess practical public health applications, such as uncovering patient subgroups in real-world datasets.

The R code generated by ChatGPT in Fig. 6.1 demonstrates the process of applying the K-means clustering algorithm using the iris dataset. It involves several essential steps: loading the necessary libraries, preparing and scaling the data, applying K-means clustering with a specified number of clusters, visualizing the clustering results using principal component analysis (PCA), and evaluating the

```r
# Load required libraries
library(ggplot2)
library(cluster)
library(factoextra)

# Load and prepare the dataset
data(iris)
iris_data <- scale(iris[, -5])  # Remove species label and scale features

# Set seed for reproducibility
set.seed(123)

# Apply K-means clustering (3 clusters, as there are 3 iris species)
kmeans_result <- kmeans(iris_data, centers = 3, nstart = 25)

# Add cluster assignments to the original dataset
iris$Cluster <- as.factor(kmeans_result$cluster)

# Visualize clusters using fviz_cluster
fviz_cluster(kmeans_result, data = iris_data,
             geom = "point", ellipse.type = "norm",
             ggtheme = theme_minimal())

# Evaluate clustering performance with contingency table
table(iris$Species, iris$Cluster)
```

Fig. 6.1 R code generated by ChatGPT to perform the K-means algorithm

results by comparing assigned clusters to known species labels. This unsupervised learning workflow enhances clarity, reproducibility, and interpretability, making it especially useful for public health professionals exploring subgroup patterns or segmenting populations based on multivariate data without relying on predefined labels.

By using a prompt such as "Provide explanations about what the K-means clustering code was doing in RStudio," ChatGPT can explain in detail each step in the workflow, including data preparation, clustering execution, visualization, and evaluation—helping users understand how unsupervised learning identifies patterns and groups within the dataset.

Following the iris example depicted in Fig. 6.2, the K-means clustering algorithm can also be applied to Electronic Health Records (EHR) to identify naturally occurring subgroups among patients based on clinical features. Unlike K-Nearest Neighbors, which relies on labeled training data, K-means is an unsupervised method that does not require predefined categories or risk labels. Instead, it partitions patients into clusters based solely on similarities in their attributes—such as age, cholesterol levels, blood pressure, BMI, and glucose levels.

For example, K-means may reveal that patients form three distinct clusters characterized by different health profiles. One cluster may consist of younger individuals with healthy metabolic indicators, another might include middle-aged patients with moderate risks, and a third could contain older adults with multiple chronic conditions. These clusters help public health professionals identify target groups for intervention without needing labeled outcome data in advance. Step 6 in Fig. 6.2 will result in the graph that is shown in Fig. 6.3:

Because K-means detects patterns directly from the structure of the data, it is especially valuable for exploratory analysis, hypothesis generation, and segmenting populations for tailored healthcare strategies. Step 7 in Fig. 6.2 produces a contingency table. Off diagonals are incorrect predictions. Table 6.1 shows that 11 Versicolor and 14 Virginica were incorrectly predicted:

Hierarchical Clustering

Hierarchical clustering is an unsupervised machine learning technique that builds a multilevel hierarchy of clusters by either successively merging smaller clusters (agglomerative approach) or successively splitting larger ones (divisive approach). In public health, hierarchical clustering is especially valuable for revealing nested subgroup structures, such as classifying patients by clinical risk profiles, genetic markers, or behavioral patterns, without requiring any predefined number of groups (Ward Jr., 1963).

Unlike K-means, which requires the number of clusters (k) to be specified in advance, hierarchical clustering does not need an initial cluster count. Instead, it constructs a dendrogram—a tree-like diagram—that visually represents the process of cluster merging or splitting. Researchers can "cut" the dendrogram at different levels to explore various subgroup structures.

1. Load Required Libraries

r Copy Edit

```r
library(ggplot2)
library(cluster)
library(factoextra)
```

These libraries are loaded to:

- Support clustering operations (`cluster`)
- Visualize results (`factoextra`)
- Enhance plotting options (`ggplot2`)

2. Load and Prepare the Dataset

r Copy Edit

```r
data(iris)
iris_data <- scale(iris[, -5])
```

- Loads the `iris` dataset.
- Removes the `Species` column (i.e., the true labels), since clustering is unsupervised.
- Scales the features so each variable contributes equally to distance computations.

3. Set Seed for Reproducibility

r Copy Edit

```r
set.seed(123)
```

Ensures that the clustering results are reproducible each time the script is run.

Fig. 6.2 Explanations generated by ChatGPT to explain how the K-means algorithm is performed in RStudio

The most common form, agglomerative hierarchical clustering, begins with each observation as its own cluster and then:

1. Computes pairwise distances (usually using Euclidean distance),
2. Merges the two closest clusters based on a linkage criterion (e.g., single, complete, or average linkage),
3. Repeats until all data points are merged into one cluster.

4. Apply K-Means Clustering

r

Copy Edit

```r
kmeans_result <- kmeans(iris_data, centers = 3, nstart = 25)
```

- Runs the K-means algorithm with **3 clusters** (because there are 3 species in the original dataset).
- `nstart = 25` tells R to try 25 different random initial cluster assignments and choose the best one based on the lowest total within-cluster sum of squares.

5. Add Cluster Assignments

r

Copy Edit

```r
iris$Cluster <- as.factor(kmeans_result$cluster)
```

Appends the clustering result to the original `iris` dataset for comparison or visualization.

6. Visualize Clusters

r

Copy Edit

```r
fviz_cluster(kmeans_result, data = iris_data,
             geom = "point", ellipse.type = "norm",
             ggtheme = theme_minimal())
```

- `fviz_cluster()` visualizes the clustered data in 2D.
- Points are plotted and grouped by assigned cluster with normal distribution ellipses around them.
- The `theme_minimal()` gives a clean, simple plot appearance.

7. Evaluate with Contingency Table

r

Copy Edit

```r
table(iris$Species, iris$Cluster)
```

- Compares the actual species labels with the cluster assignments.
- Helps assess how well the unsupervised clusters align with the true species groups, even though the algorithm had no access to these labels.

Fig. 6.2 (continued)

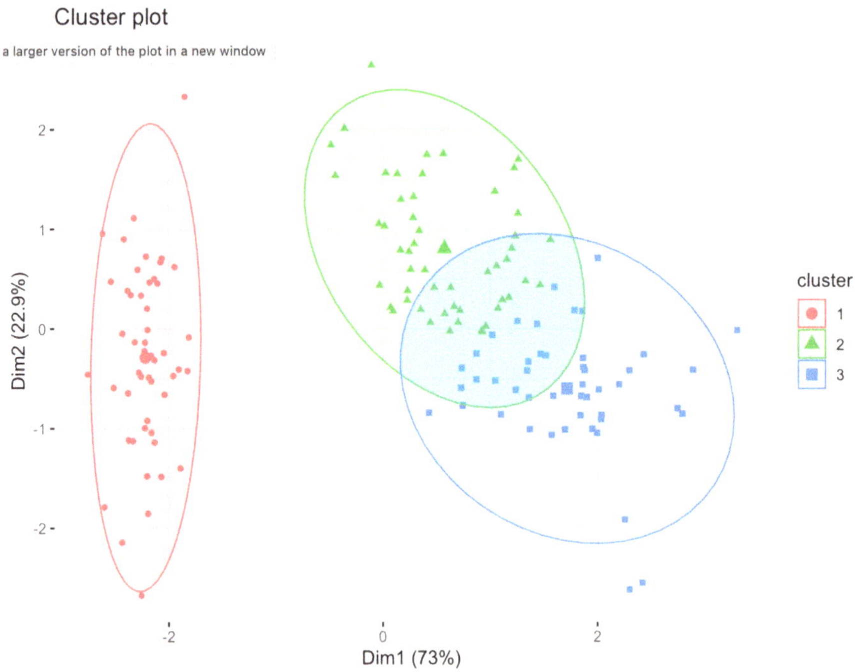

Fig. 6.3 Clusters generated by the K-means algorithm in RStudio

Table 6.1 A contingency table produced by the K-means algorithm in RStudio

	1	2	3
Setosa	50	0	0
Versicolor	0	39	11
Virginica	0	14	36

This method is particularly effective for understanding the relationships between individuals or variables in a dataset, identifying meaningful groupings, and performing exploratory analyses in high-dimensional healthcare data. More formally, hierarchical clustering involves distance computations similar to the Euclidean distance used in KNN and K-means algorithms. Mathematically:

$$d(x, y) = \sqrt{\sum_{i=1}^{n} (x_i - y_i)^2}$$

where:

- $d(x, y)$ is the Euclidean distance between observations x and y,
- x_i and y_i represent the respective values of feature i in the observations,
- n is the number of features.

In hierarchical clustering, once the distance is computed, clusters are merged based on a linkage criterion, such as single linkage, complete linkage, or average linkage. These linkage criteria guide the hierarchical clustering process by determining which clusters should be joined at each step, ultimately forming the hierarchical structure (also called dendrogram in ML) for exploration and analysis.

USArrests Dataset Example

To illustrate hierarchical clustering, we use the built-in R dataset `USArrests`. This dataset includes four numeric variables for each US state: murder, assault, urban population, and rape. Although no class labels exist, hierarchical clustering can help identify natural groupings based on crime patterns.

A user might prompt ChatGPT as follows: "Provide R code to apply hierarchical clustering on the `USArrests` dataset, including visualization and interpretation." Figure 6.4 presents a full R example that includes scaling, computing distances, performing hierarchical clustering, and visualizing results:

The R code generated by ChatGPT, as shown in Fig. 6.4, demonstrates how to apply **hierarchical clustering** using the built-in USArrests dataset. The workflow includes key steps: loading and scaling the data, calculating a distance matrix using Euclidean distance, performing hierarchical clustering using the complete linkage method, and visualizing the results through a dendrogram and cluster plots.

Unlike K-means, hierarchical clustering does not require pre-specifying the number of clusters. Hierarchical cluster analysis (HCA), also known as hierarchical clustering, is a popular method for cluster analysis in big data research and data mining aiming to establish a hierarchy of clusters (Zhang et al., 2017). Instead, it builds a tree (dendrogram) that represents nested groupings of data points based on similarity. This allows users to visually explore the data's structure and decide on the number of meaningful clusters by "cutting" the dendrogram at a chosen height.

This unsupervised learning approach is valuable for public health professionals aiming to identify natural groupings in multivariate data—such as crime patterns, disease prevalence, or behavioral risk factors—without relying on pre-labeled categories. Hierarchical clustering methods have been used to identify groups of countries with similar labor market regulations, allowing analysis of important associations between socioeconomic conditions and public health that would remain hidden from traditional indicators like Gross National Product (Loftus et al., 2022). It supports exploratory data analysis and pattern recognition in scenarios where group boundaries are unknown or ambiguous.

By using a prompt such as "Explain the hierarchical clustering code in R," ChatGPT can guide users through each phase of the analysis, including data standardization, distance computation, clustering method selection, and result interpretation—enhancing transparency, reproducibility, and practical understanding of unsupervised learning in public health contexts.

```r
r                                                          Copy  Edit

# Libraries
# install.packages(c("cluster", "factoextra"))  # if needed
library(cluster)
library(factoextra)

# Data and scaled_data
data("USArrests")
data <- na.omit(USArrests)
scaled_data <- scale(data)

# Distance matrix
dist_matrix <- dist(scaled_data, method = "euclidean")

# Hierarchical clustering (complete linkage)
hc_complete <- hclust(dist_matrix, method = "complete")

# Dendrogram
plot(hc_complete,
     main = "USArrests – Hierarchical Clustering (complete linkage)",
     xlab = "", sub = "", cex = 0.6)

# Rectangles to show k clusters
k <- 3
rect.hclust(hc_complete, k = k, border = "red")

# Cluster visualization with factoextra
clusters <- cutree(hc_complete, k = k)
fviz_cluster(
  list(data = scaled_data, cluster = clusters),
  main = sprintf("USArrests – Cluster Plot (k = %d)", k),
  ellipse.type = "t",
  repel = TRUE
)
```

Fig. 6.4 R code generated by ChatGPT to perform the hierarchical clustering algorithm

Hierarchical clustering is a valuable tool in public health for identifying natural groupings within complex datasets, such as Electronic Health Records (EHR). Unlike supervised methods, it does not require predefined labels or risk categories. Instead, it organizes individuals into clusters based on similarities in characteristics like age, blood pressure, and other health indicators. The dendrogram in the R code (see Fig. 6.5) will result in the dendrogram depicted in Fig. 6.6:

This approach helps public health professionals explore hidden patterns, generate hypotheses, and define patient subgroups for targeted interventions—especially when clear categories are not available. Because it builds a tree-like structure of relationships, hierarchical clustering is ideal for understanding how groups evolve and relate to one another in population health data.

Libraries

- `cluster` provides algorithms and diagnostics for clustering.
- `factoextra` offers convenient, publication-ready visualizations (dendrograms, cluster plots).
- Managerial relevance: these tools help turn raw data into understandable segments for decision making (e.g., regional strategy, resource allocation).

Data and scaling

r Copy Edit

```r
data("USArrests")
data <- na.omit(USArrests)
scaled_data <- scale(data)
```

- Loads the **USArrests** dataset (crime rates and urbanization by U.S. state).
- Removes any rows with missing values to avoid errors.
- Standardizes each variable (mean 0, SD 1) so features measured on different scales contribute equally.
- Why scale: without scaling, variables with larger numeric ranges would dominate distance calculations and bias the clustering.

Distance matrix

r Copy Edit

```r
dist_matrix <- dist(scaled_data, method = "euclidean")
```

- Computes pairwise **Euclidean distances** between states on the standardized features.
- This captures how similar or dissimilar states are in a multivariate sense.
- Interpretation: smaller distance = more similar crime/urban profiles.

Fig. 6.5 Explanations generated by ChatGPT to explain how the hierarchical clustering algorithm is performed in RStudio

RStudio can also produce two-dimensional plots to represent the clusters by colors. The "fviz_cluster" command in R code (see Fig. 6.5) will produce three clusters in a Cluster Plot, as depicted in Fig. 6.7:

Principal Component Analysis (PCA)

Principal Component Analysis (PCA) is the **final unsupervised machine learning model introduced in this chapter**. Unlike clustering methods that form groups of similar observations, PCA is primarily used for **dimensionality reduction**. PCA reduces the dimensionality of complex datasets by creating new variables called components that retain the majority of the original data's variability (Jolliffe, 2002). It transforms a dataset with many correlated variables into a smaller set of

Hierarchical clustering (complete linkage)

r Copy Edit

```r
hc_complete <- hclust(dist_matrix, method = "complete")
```

- Builds a hierarchy (tree) by iteratively joining the **most similar** clusters, using **complete linkage** (distance between clusters = the farthest pair of points across clusters).
- Complete linkage tends to create compact, evenly sized clusters and is conservative about merging dissimilar points.
- Managerial trade-off: more compact clusters improve interpretability for segmentation; different linkage choices can yield different group structures.

Dendrogram

r Copy Edit

```r
plot(hc_complete, main = "USArrests – Hierarchical Clustering (complete linkage)",
     xlab = "", sub = "", cex = 0.6)
```

- Visualizes the clustering as a tree. Each leaf is a state; branches show which states or clusters merged and at what dissimilarity.
- Reading the plot: lower merge height = more similar; higher merge height = more dissimilar.

Choosing a number of clusters and drawing rectangles

r Copy Edit

```r
k <- 3
rect.hclust(hc_complete, k = k, border = "red")
```

- Selects **k = 3** clusters by "cutting" the dendrogram at a chosen height, then outlines them on the plot.
- How to choose k: look for large vertical gaps in the dendrogram (big jumps in merge height), domain logic (e.g., three market segments), or validation metrics (e.g., silhouette).

Cluster visualization (PCA projection)

r Copy Edit

```r
clusters <- cutree(hc_complete, k = k)
fviz_cluster(
  list(data = scaled_data, cluster = clusters),
  main = sprintf("USArrests – Cluster Plot (k = %d)", k),
  ellipse.type = "t",
  repel = TRUE
)
```

- `cutree()` assigns each state to one of the k clusters.
- `fviz_cluster()` projects the high-dimensional data into two principal components for a 2D plot and colors points by cluster, with optional ellipses around groups.
- Interpretation: clusters that are well separated on the plot suggest distinct profiles (e.g., states with similar crime rates and urbanization). Overlap suggests fuzzier boundaries and potential need to revisit k or linkage.

Fig. 6.5 (continued)

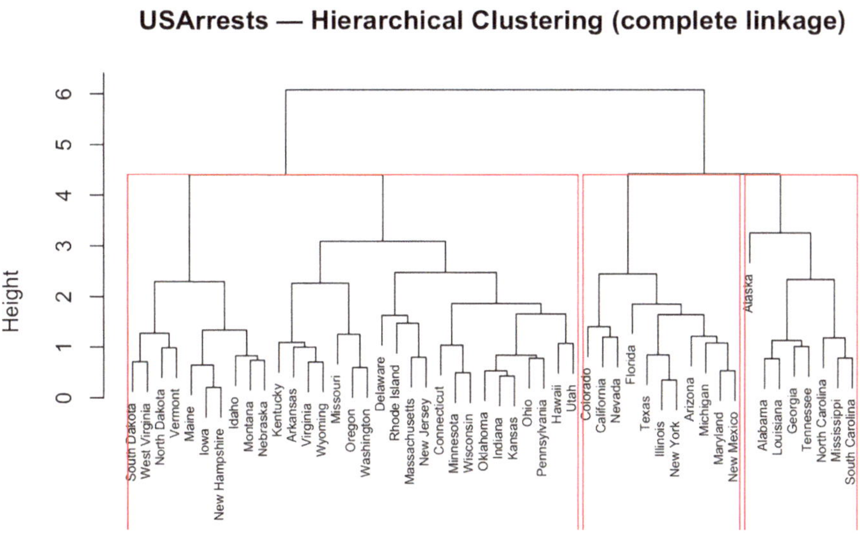

Fig. 6.6 A dendrogram generated by the hierarchical algorithm in RStudio

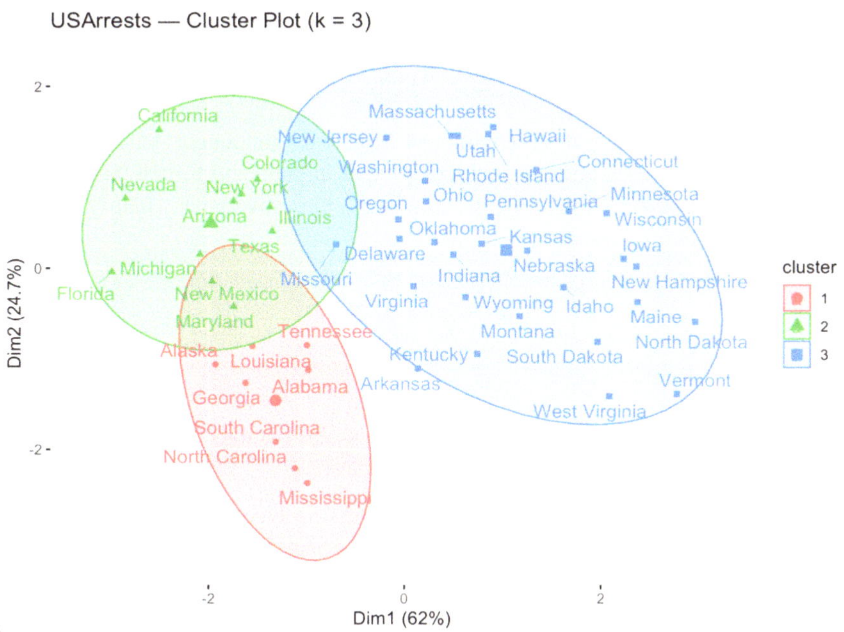

Fig. 6.7 Clusters generated by the hierarchical algorithm in RStudio

uncorrelated variables—called **principal components**—that retain most of the original data's variation.

In public health research, PCA is especially useful for analyzing **high-dimensional datasets**—such as large-scale surveys, genomics, or electronic health records—by revealing the latent structure of the data without requiring labeled outcomes or predefined categories. PCA can also be a useful statistical method for constructing socioeconomic status (SES) measures and identifying variations across different community areas (Friesen et al., 2016; Wu et al., 2016).

The typical PCA process involves:

1. Standardizing the data to give each variable equal weight,
2. Computing the covariance matrix to capture relationships between variables,
3. Deriving principal components as new axes that maximize variance,
4. Selecting components that explain the majority of total variance.

PCA helps public health professionals:

- Visualize complex datasets in two or three dimensions,
- Identify latent patterns such as disease progression or social determinants of health,
- Reduce noise or redundancy, making data easier to interpret and use in subsequent models.

As a final tool in the suite of unsupervised learning methods covered in this chapter, PCA complements clustering approaches by offering a *continuous, rather than categorical,* perspective on data structure. It is especially valuable when preparing data for further modeling or when exploring multivariate relationships across public health domains.

Below is the formulaic representation of Principal Component Analysis (PCA), along with a brief explanation of each component in plain and formal language:

Covariance matrix—First, PCA computes the covariance matrix of the standardized data:

$$\mathbf{C} = \frac{1}{n-1}\mathbf{X}^T\mathbf{X}$$

where:

- **X:** The $n \times p$ standardized data matrix (with n observations and p variables).
- **C:** The $p \times p$ covariance matrix of the variables.

Eigen Decomposition—Second, PCA performs an eigen decomposition of the covariance matrix:

$$\mathbf{C}\mathbf{v}_i = \lambda_i \mathbf{v}_i$$

where:

- $\boldsymbol{\lambda_i v_i}$**:** The eigenvalue associated with the i-th principal component (represents the amount of variance explained)
- $\mathbf{v_i}$**:** The eigenvector (principal axis or direction) corresponding to λ_i

Principal Component Scores—Finally, to project the original data onto the new axes:

$$\mathbf{z} = \mathbf{XV}$$

where:

- **Z:** The matrix of principal component scores (transformed data in the new coordinate system).
- **V:** The matrix of eigenvectors (columns are the principal components).

Interpretation in Public Health Context—Each row in Z is a transformed observation, now described by principal component**s** instead of original variables. The first few components usually capture the dominant patterns in the data (e.g., variations in patient risk profiles or regional health disparities), which can then be used for visualization, interpretation, or further analysis.

USArrests Dataset Example: Principal Component Analysis (PCA)

To illustrate Principal Component Analysis (PCA), we use the built-in R dataset USArrests. This dataset includes four numeric variables for each US state: **Murder**, **Assault**, **UrbanPop**, and **Rape**. These variables represent different types of crime rates and demographic factors across states. Although no class labels are available, PCA can help reduce the dimensionality of the data while preserving the most important variance patterns.

A user might prompt ChatGPT as: "Provide R code to apply PCA on the USArrests dataset, including visualization and interpretation." Figure 6.8 shows a complete R example that performs PCA, visualizes the results, and helps interpret the relationships between states and variables:

The R code generated by ChatGPT above demonstrates how to apply PCA using the built-in USArrests dataset. The workflow includes essential steps: loading and scaling the data, computing principal components, and visualizing the results through a scree plot and a biplot.

Unlike clustering methods that aim to group similar observations, PCA focuses on *dimensionality reduction* by identifying new axes (principal components) that capture the most variance in the data. This technique transforms a high-dimensional

```r
r                                                          Copy  Edit

# Install if needed:
# install.packages("factoextra")

library(datasets)
library(factoextra)

# load data and scale
data("USArrests")
scaled_data <- scale(USArrests)

# PCA
pca_result <- prcomp(scaled_data, center = FALSE, scale. = FALSE)

# variance explained (eigenvalues)
fviz_eig(pca_result, addlabels = TRUE, main = "USArrests – PCA: Variance E

# biplot
fviz_pca_biplot(
  pca_result,
  repel = TRUE,
  title = "USArrests – PCA Biplot (scaled)"
)
```

Fig. 6.8 R code generated by ChatGPT to perform the PCA algorithm

dataset into a smaller number of interpretable dimensions without requiring predefined categories or outcomes.

PCA is widely used in exploratory data analysis, particularly in high-dimensional settings common in public health and epidemiological studies. It helps researchers uncover dominant patterns—such as crime profiles across US states—by projecting complex data onto a simpler structure. The biplot enables users to examine how states relate to each other and to specific crime indicators (e.g., murder or assault rates).

In public health applications, PCA can reveal underlying structures in multivariate datasets such as health behaviors, environmental exposures, or chronic disease indicators. This supports tasks such as:

(a) Identifying patterns or gradients across geographic regions,
(b) Reducing redundancy in health surveillance data,
(c) Preparing variables for downstream analysis (e.g., clustering or regression).

As the final unsupervised method introduced in this chapter, PCA complements clustering techniques by offering a *continuous, geometry-based view* of data structure that enhances interpretability and supports data-driven decision-making.

By using a prompt such as "Explain the PCA code in R," ChatGPT can guide users through each phase of the analysis, including data standardization, computation of principal components, variance interpretation, and visualization through scree plots and biplots. This supports greater transparency, reproducibility, and practical understanding of unsupervised learning in public health contexts—particularly when exploring complex, high-dimensional datasets without predefined labels.

In public health, Principal Component Analysis (PCA) can be effectively applied to high-dimensional data sources such as Electronic Health Records (EHRs), surveys, or behavioral datasets to uncover dominant patterns across multiple variables—without relying on labeled outcomes. Secondary use of electronic health records (EHRs) can improve clinical research and better inform decision-making. However, EHR may contain a large number of interrelated variables, leading to multicollinearity issues in regression analysis (Zhang & Castello, 2017). Unlike supervised methods, PCA is an unsupervised technique that reduces data complexity by transforming correlated variables (e.g., age, cholesterol, BMI, and blood pressure) into a smaller set of uncorrelated principal components that explain most of the variance in the data.

For example, PCA may reveal that the first component captures overall cardiometabolic risk, while the second component reflects differences in lifestyle factors or social determinants. Each patient or population group can then be positioned along these new dimensions, enabling researchers to detect hidden gradients of risk or health status. PCA applies an orthogonal transformation to turn potentially correlated variables into a new set of linearly independent variables, known as principal components. The number of these components is equal to or fewer than the original variables in the dataset (Miotto et al., 2016). The R code (see Fig. 6.9) lists the variance explained (eigenvalues) as a graph in Fig. 6.10:

PCA results allow public health professionals to:

- Explore multivariate trends,
- Visualize complex data in two or three dimensions,
- Identify emerging subgroups for further investigation or intervention,
- And reduce redundancy for use in predictive models.

PCA is especially useful during the exploratory phase of analysis, for hypothesis generation, and for preparing large datasets for downstream modeling or clustering—offering a more interpretable and data-driven approach to understanding health complexity in diverse populations. The R code (see Fig. 6.10) also produces a PCA biplot, as shown in Fig. 6.11:

1. Load libraries

- `datasets` provides built-in datasets (including `USArrests`).
- `factoextra` adds high-quality PCA visualizations (`fviz_eig()`, `fviz_pca_biplot()`).
- Management lens: these tools turn complex multivariate data into simple visuals for segmentation and strategic comparisons.

2. Load and standardize the data

r Copy Edit

```r
data("USArrests")
scaled_data <- scale(USArrests)
```

- `USArrests` contains crime and urbanization measures by U.S. state, on different scales.
- `scale()` standardizes each variable (mean 0, SD 1) so no single measure dominates because of its units.
- Why this matters: fair comparison across variables improves pattern detection and reduces bias in component estimates.

Fig. 6.9 Explanations generated by ChatGPT regarding how the PCA algorithm is performed in RStudio

Comparison of Unsupervised Learning Models

Unsupervised learning models are essential tools in public health and management research for exploring patterns, segmenting populations, and reducing data complexity—without requiring labeled outcome variables. These models vary in method, interpretation, and purpose. Table 6.2 summarizes the key similarities and differences among three foundational unsupervised learning models, highlighting their typical use cases and R dataset examples.

Summary

All three models share a fundamental goal: to extract insights from unlabeled, multivariate data in a way that reveals hidden structure and supports decision-making. One of the most important unsupervised learning techniques is clustering, which is the process of partitioning a set of data points according to some measure of similarity (e.g., distance). The goal of clustering is to reveal subgroups within heterogeneous data such that each individual cluster exhibits meaningful patterns

3. Run PCA

r Copy Edit

```
pca_result <- prcomp(scaled_data, center = FALSE, scale. = FALSE)
```

- `prcomp()` computes principal components on the already standardized matrix.
- `center = FALSE, scale. = FALSE` is deliberate: we **already** centered and scaled with `scale()`. Re-doing it would distort results.

4. Variance explained (eigenvalues) plot

r Copy Edit

```
fviz_eig(pca_result, addlabels = TRUE, main = "USArrests – PCA: Variance E
```

- Shows each component's share of total variance and the cumulative curve.
- Use this to choose how many components to keep (e.g., "elbow" point or a threshold like 80–90% cumulative variance).
- Managerial takeaway: fewer components = simpler dashboards/models with minimal information loss.

5. PCA biplot

r Copy Edit

```
fviz_pca_biplot(
  pca_result,
  repel = TRUE,
  title = "USArrests – PCA Biplot (scaled)"
)
```

- Plots states (points) in the first two principal components and overlays variable loadings (arrows).
- Interpreting the biplot:
  - **Points close together** → states with **similar profiles** across variables.
  - **Arrow direction** → the direction of increase for a variable; **length** ~ contribution to these components.
  - **Angle between arrows** → correlation (small angle = positive correlation; ~180° = negative).
  - **Projection of a point on an arrow** ≈ relative value of that variable for the state.
- Management use: quickly see groups of states with comparable risk patterns, identify drivers (arrows), and brief stakeholders with an intuitive map.

Fig. 6.9 (continued)

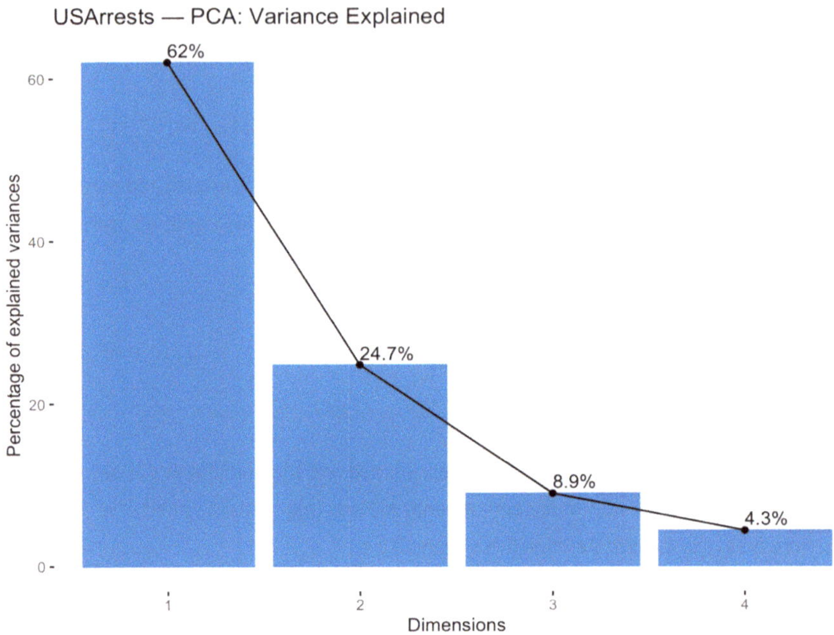

Fig. 6.10 Variance explained by eigenvalue in the PCA algorithm in RStudio

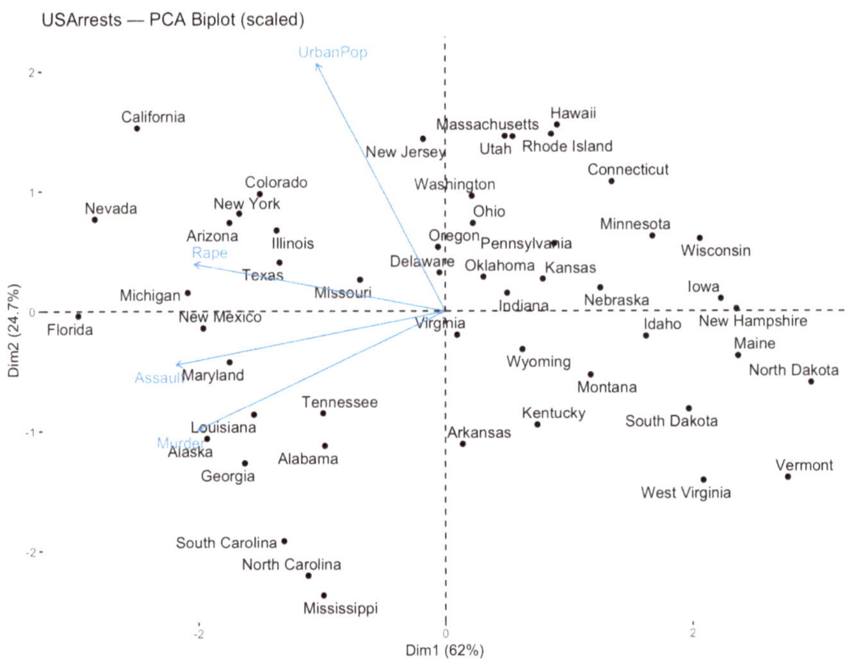

Fig. 6.11 Clusters generated by the PCA algorithm in RStudio

Table 6.2 Comparison of 3 unsupervised learning models: K-means clustering, hierarchical clustering, and principal component analysis (PCA)

Model	Key features	Purpose / typical use	Illustrative dataset	Similarities	Differences
K-Means clustering	Centroid-based; partitions data into *k* clusters by minimizing within-cluster variance	Identifying subgroups in population data based on health profiles	Iris	No labels required; exploratory pattern discovery	Requires pre-specifying number of clusters (*k*); sensitive to scaling
Hierarchical clustering	Builds tree-like structure (dendrogram); uses distance and linkage criteria	Revealing nested relationships (e.g., by geography or comorbidity)	USArrests	No predefined labels; reveals structure in multivariate data	No need to predefine number of clusters; supports visual "cutting"
Principal component analysis (PCA)	Linear transformation; projects data to lower dimensions while preserving variance	Reducing complexity, identifying principal risk dimensions	USArrests	Used for exploratory analysis, no labels needed	Does not cluster data directly; reveals variance structure, not groups

(Alashwal et al., 2019). They are especially suited for exploratory data analysis, hypothesis generation, and preprocessing for further modeling or intervention planning.

However, each model differs in output and analytical focus. K-means produces clear group membership for each observation, while hierarchical clustering uncovers nested subgroupings and relationships. In contrast, PCA provides continuous dimensions (principal components) that summarize variation, useful for visualizing and simplifying complex datasets.

Unsupervised machine learning, as opposed to supervised learning, has shown promise in identifying novel patterns and relations from EHRs without using human created labels (Wang et al., 2020). K-means is particularly useful for identifying latent subgroups in patient or population data, such as behavioral or metabolic risk clusters. Hierarchical clustering can help uncover multilevel patterns in social determinants, regional disparities, or comorbidities by revealing the nested structure of relationships within health data. Meanwhile, PCA aids in simplifying high-dimensional datasets like EHRs or health surveys, making patterns more interpretable and visual by reducing the complexity of multivariate information into comprehensible components.

Each method offers unique advantages. When selecting an approach, researchers should consider the structure of their data, their analytical goals (e.g., segmentation vs. simplification), and how results will inform public health strategies or interventions.

Together, these unsupervised models provide a foundational toolkit for understanding patterns in population health without relying on pre-existing labels or categories.

Discussion Questions

1. How can clustering methods like K-means or hierarchical clustering be applied to uncover patterns in public health or management data?
2. What are the key differences between K-means clustering and hierarchical clustering, and how do these differences influence their suitability for different types of datasets?
3. In the absence of labeled outcomes, what strategies can be used to evaluate the effectiveness of an unsupervised learning model?
4. What ethical concerns should be considered when using unsupervised learning to segment populations or group individuals in applied settings?
5. How does dimensionality reduction (e.g., PCA) support or hinder the interpretation of complex datasets in public health and management research?

References

Alashwal, H., El Halaby, M., Crouse, J. J., Abdalla, A., & Moustafa, A. A. (2019). The application of unsupervised clustering methods to Alzheimer's disease. *Frontiers in Computational Neuroscience, 13*, 31. https://doi.org/10.3389/fncom.2019.00031. PMID: 31178711; PMCID: PMC6543980. https://pmc.ncbi.nlm.nih.gov/articles/PMC6543980/

Bishop, C. M. (2006). *Pattern recognition and machine learning*. Springer. https://www.springer.com/gp/book/9780387310732

Friesen, C. E., Seliske, P., & Papadopoulos, A. (2016). Using principal component analysis to identify priority neighbourhoods for health services delivery by ranking socioeconomic status. *Online Journal of Public Health Informatics, 8*(2), e192. https://doi.org/10.5210/ojphi.v8i2.6733

Hastie, T., Tibshirani, R., & Friedman, J. (2009). *The elements of statistical learning: Data mining, inference, and prediction* (2nd ed.). Springer. https://web.stanford.edu/~hastie/ElemStatLearn/

Hennig, C. (2007). Cluster-wise assessment of cluster stability. *Computational Statistics & Data Analysis, 52*(1), 258–271. https://doi.org/10.1016/j.csda.2006.11.025

Hotelling, H. (1933). Analysis of a complex of statistical variables into principal components. *Journal of Educational Psychology, 24*(6), 417–441. https://doi.org/10.1037/h0071325

Jain, A. K. (2010). Data clustering: 50 years beyond K-means. *Pattern Recognition Letters, 31*(8), 651–666. https://doi.org/10.1016/j.patrec.2009.09.011

Johnson, S. C. (1967). Hierarchical clustering schemes. *Psychometrika, 32*(3), 241–254. https://doi.org/10.1007/BF02289588

Jolliffe, I. T. (2002). *Principal component analysis* (2nd ed.). Springer. https://link.springer.com/book/10.1007/b98835

Likas, A., Vlassis, N., & Verbeek, J. J. (2003). The global k-means clustering algorithm. *Pattern Recognition, 36*(2), 451–461. https://doi.org/10.1016/S0031-3203(02)00060-2

Loftus, T. J., Shickel, B., Balch, J. A., Tighe, P. J., Abbott, K. L., Fazzone, B., Anderson, E. M., Rozowsky, J., Ozrazgat-Baslanti, T., Ren, Y., Berceli, S. A., Hogan, W. R., Efron, P. A., Moorman, J. R., Rashidi, P., Upchurch, G. R., Jr., & Bihorac, A. (2022). Phenotype clustering in health care: A narrative review for clinicians. *Frontiers in Artificial Intelligence, 5*, 842306.

https://doi.org/10.3389/frai.2022.842306. https://www.frontiersin.org/journals/artificial-intelligence/articles/10.3389/frai.2022.842306/full

MacQueen, J. (1967). Some methods for classification and analysis of multivariate observations. In *Proceedings of the fifth Berkeley symposium on mathematical statistics and probability* (Vol. 1, pp. 281–297). University of California Press. https://projecteuclid.org/euclid.bsmsp/1200512992

Miotto, R., Li, L., Kidd, B. A., & Dudley, J. T. (2016). Deep patient: An unsupervised representation to predict the future of patients from the electronic health records. *Scientific Reports, 6*(1), 1–10. https://doi.org/10.1038/srep26094

Pearson, K. (1901). On lines and planes of closest fit to systems of points in space. *The London, Edinburgh, and Dublin Philosophical Magazine and Journal of Science, 2*(11), 559–572. https://doi.org/10.1080/14786440109462720

Rajkomar, A., Oren, E., Chen, K., Dai, A. M., Hajaj, N., Hardt, M., et al. (2018). Scalable and accurate deep learning with electronic health records. *npj Digital Medicine, 1*(1), 1–10. https://doi.org/10.1038/s41746-018-0029-1

Rousseeuw, P. J. (1987). Silhouettes: A graphical aid to the interpretation and validation of cluster analysis. *Journal of Computational and Applied Mathematics, 20*, 53–65. https://doi.org/10.1016/0377-0427(87)90125-7

Tomar, D., & Agarwal, S. (2013). A survey on data mining approaches for healthcare. *International Journal of Bio-Science and Bio-Technology, 5*(5), 241–266. https://doi.org/10.14257/ijbsbt.2013.5.5.25

Wang, Y., Zhao, Y., Therneau, T. M., Atkinson, E. J., Tafti, A. P., Zhang, N., Amin, S., Limper, A. H., Khosla, S., & Liu, H. (2020). Unsupervised machine learning for the discovery of latent disease clusters and patient subgroups using electronic health records. *Journal of Biomedical Informatics, 102*, 103364. ISSN 1532-0464. https://doi.org/10.1016/j.jbi.2019.103364

Ward, J. H., Jr. (1963). Hierarchical grouping to optimize an objective function. *Journal of the American Statistical Association, 58*(301), 236–244. https://doi.org/10.1080/01621459.1963.10500845

Wu, X., Kirk, S. F., Ohinmaa, A., & Veugelers, P. (2016). Health behaviours, body weight and self-esteem among grade five students in Canada. *Springerplus, 5*(1), 1099. https://doi.org/10.1186/s40064-016-2744-x

Zhang, Z., & Castelló, A. (2017). Principal components analysis in clinical studies. *Annals of Translational Medicine, 5*(17), 351. https://doi.org/10.21037/atm.2017.07.12. PMID: 28936445; PMCID: PMC5599285. https://www.ncbi.nlm.nih.gov/pmc/articles/PMC5599285/

Zhang, Z., Murtagh, F., Van Poucke, S., Lin, S., & Lan, P. (2017). Hierarchical cluster analysis in clinical research with heterogeneous study population: Highlighting its visualization with R. *Annals of Translational Medicine, 5*(4), 75. https://doi.org/10.21037/atm.2017.02.05. PMID: 28275620; PMCID: PMC5337204. https://pubmed.ncbi.nlm.nih.gov/28275620/

Chapter 7
Advanced Machine Learning Models

Learning Objectives

By the end of this chapter, advanced readers will be able to:

1. **Understand** and **implement** advanced ML models using R or RStudio.
2. **Use** given datasets to grasp the core mathematical ideas behind each technique.
3. **Use** AI tools like ChatGPT to support self-directed learning and problem-solving.
4. **Interpret** the outputs of advanced machine learning models.
5. **Identify** common challenges and best practices when applying advanced machine learning models to real-world public health problems.

Introduction

This chapter is designed for readers who already have a basic understanding of machine learning concepts and are ready to engage with more advanced models and analytical techniques. If you are new to machine learning, you may choose to skip this chapter for now and revisit it after gaining familiarity with fundamental models and methods presented in earlier chapters. The focus here is on advanced machine learning models, including Support Vector Machine (SVM), Gradient Boosting, Deep Learning, and Natural Language Processing (NLP), all within the context of public health research (Beam & Kohane, 2018).

For clarity and accessibility, we illustrate the mathematical computations of each model using a simple dataset consisting of 10 observations and 3 variables. This approach allows readers to follow the calculations step by step without being overwhelmed by complex data (James et al., 2021). In addition, we demonstrate how generative AI tools such as ChatGPT can be used to assist in the learning

---

Supplementary Information The online version contains supplementary material available at https://doi.org/10.1007/978-3-032-08677-8_7.

R. Leung, *Leveraging GenAI for Machine Learning Education in Public Health*,
https://doi.org/10.1007/978-3-032-08677-8_7

process. For example, students can prompt ChatGPT to generate code, explain model outputs, or clarify mathematical reasoning at each stage of model development (Kasneci et al., 2023).

The integration of advanced machine learning techniques in public health research has shown remarkable promise in addressing complex epidemiological challenges, from predicting disease outbreaks to personalizing treatment strategies (Rajkomar et al., 2019). These sophisticated algorithms can identify subtle patterns in large-scale health datasets that traditional statistical methods might miss, enabling more precise risk stratification and intervention targeting. However, the successful application of these methods requires not only technical proficiency but also a deep understanding of their theoretical foundations, assumptions, and limitations within the public health context (Chen & Asch, 2017).

Unlike previous chapters, which used built-in R datasets directly as examples to demonstrate machine learning applications in public health, this chapter adopts a different approach. Here, we use a simulated dataset with a small number of observations and variables to illustrate the mathematical foundations of advanced models. This approach enables readers to follow step-by-step computations for each method, making the underlying concepts clearer without the added complexity of larger or less structured datasets. By focusing on simplified data, the essential logic and calculations of each advanced machine learning model are made more transparent and accessible.

Simulating a Simple Dataset in R with ChatGPT Assistance

(a) Prompting ChatGPT

Sample Prompt *I would like to create a simple dataset in R with 100 observations and 5 variables. The first variable should be a numeric variable age, the second variable should be a categorical variable with two categories gender, and the third variable should be a continuous outcome variable blood pressure, and fourth variable is risk with 2 categories high and low. Also a qualitative text variable doctors_notes for clinical notes. Please provide R code to generate this data frame with random values.*

(b) ChatGPT's Suggested R Code

As depicted in Fig. 7.1, the following results return in ChatGPT:

Simulated Data—Use the Copy icon on the upper right in the output above, and we can paste the codes in RStudio. Then, in RStudio, we can highlight the entire code and run it. The simulated data will be created. Figure 7.2 illustrates the results:

```r
r                                                    Copy  Edit

set.seed(123) # For reproducibility

n <- 100

age <- sample(20:60, n, replace = TRUE)
gender <- sample(c("Male", "Female"), n, replace = TRUE)
blood_pressure <- round(rnorm(n, mean = 120, sd = 15), 1)
risk <- ifelse((age > 45 & blood_pressure > 130) | blood_pressure > 140, "high", "low")

notes_samples <- c(
  "Patient reports chest pain and shortness of breath.",
  "Routine checkup. No significant complaints.",
  "Elevated blood pressure observed during visit.",
  "Patient advised to reduce salt intake.",
  "Reports frequent headaches and dizziness.",
  "No history of cardiovascular issues. Regular physical activity."
)
doctors_notes <- sample(notes_samples, n, replace = TRUE)

df <- data.frame(
  age = age,
  gender = gender,
  blood_pressure = blood_pressure,
  risk = factor(risk, levels = c("low", "high")),
  doctors_notes = doctors_notes,
  stringsAsFactors = FALSE
)

head(df, 10)
```

Fig. 7.1 R code generated by ChatGPT to create a simulated dataset with 5 variables and 100 observations

Explanation of the R Code—The following step-by-step explanations are generated by ChatGPT. Without showing the ChatGPT software interface, these steps are listed below with minimal editing:

1. set.seed(123)
   Purpose: Ensures reproducibility. When you use set.seed(), running the code multiple times will give you the same random results.
2. n < − 100
   Purpose: Sets the number of observations (rows) in your dataset to 100.
3. age < − sample(20:60, n, replace = TRUE)
   Purpose: Randomly selects 100 ages between 20 and 60 (inclusive).
   Each age can appear more than once because replace = TRUE.

df

Filter

	age	gender	blood_pressure	risk	doctors_notes
1	50	Male	123.5	low	Patient advised to reduce salt intake.
2	34	Female	121.2	low	No history of cardiovascular issues. Regular physical ...
3	33	Male	105.6	low	Patient advised to reduce salt intake.
4	22	Male	118.9	low	Reports frequent headaches and dizziness.
5	56	Male	141.7	high	Patient advised to reduce salt intake.
6	33	Male	126.8	low	No history of cardiovascular issues. Regular physical ...
7	44	Male	120.6	low	Patient reports chest pain and shortness of breath.
8	45	Male	113.7	low	Routine checkup. No significant complaints.
9	46	Male	89.2	low	Patient reports chest pain and shortness of breath.
10	24	Female	137.0	low	Routine checkup. No significant complaints.
11	46	Female	98.1	low	Elevated blood pressure observed during visit.
12	47	Female	131.1	high	Routine checkup. No significant complaints.

Fig. 7.2 First 12 observations of the simulated data

4. gender <– sample(c("Male," "Female"), n, replace = TRUE)
   Purpose: Randomly assigns each observation a gender, with equal probability of "Male" or "Female."
6. blood_pressure < – round(rnorm(n, mean = 120, sd = 15), 1)
   Purpose: Simulates 100 blood pressure values from a normal distribution with mean 120 and standard deviation 15. Values are rounded to 1 decimal place for realism.
7. risk <– ifelse((age > 45 & blood_pressure > 130) | blood_pressure > 140, "high," "low")
   Purpose: Creates a binary risk category:
   (a) "high" risk if age is above 45 and blood pressure is above 130, or if blood pressure is very high (above 140)
   (b) Otherwise, assigns "low" risk.
8. notes_samples <– c(…)
   Purpose: Defines a small set of example clinical notes (text strings) to randomly assign to each record.
9. doctors_notes <– sample(notes_samples, n, replace = TRUE)
   Purpose: For each observation, randomly assigns one of the pre-defined clinical note texts.
10. df < – data.frame(…)
    Purpose: Combines all five variables into a single structured table (data frame) named df.
    Sets risk as a factor with levels "low" and "high."
11. head(df, 10)
    Purpose: Displays the first 10 rows of your dataset for quick review.

Support Vector Machine

Support Vector Machine (SVM) is a widely used supervised machine learning algorithm for classification tasks. Unlike unsupervised algorithms such as K-means, SVM requires labeled training data. SVMs have demonstrated significant utility across diverse fields, with applications ranging from chemoinformatics and drug discovery (Rodríguez-Pérez & Bajorath, 2022) to cancer genomics research (Huang et al., 2018), making them valuable in management and public health research for distinguishing between classes—such as identifying patients at high or low risk of disease—based on observed features (e.g., age, gender, blood pressure).

SVM works by finding the optimal boundary (called a hyperplane) that best separates the classes in the feature space. The algorithm seeks to maximize the margin, which is the distance between the hyperplane and the nearest observations from each class (called support vectors). This margin maximization principle is fundamental to SVM‘s effectiveness in classification tasks (Huang et al., 2018). The key steps of SVM classification are:

1. *Map observations into a multidimensional space* defined by the predictor variables (for example, age and blood pressure).
2. *Find the hyperplane* that maximizes the margin between classes (e.g., high vs. low risk), subject to constraints that minimize classification error.
3. *Classify new observations* based on which side of the hyperplane they fall on.

Support Vector Machine (SVM) and the Simulated Dataset

The SVM (Support Vector Machine) algorithm finds the optimal boundary (called a hyperplane) that separates classes by maximizing the margin between them. Instead of selecting nearest neighbors by distance as in KNN, SVM constructs a separating line (or hyperplane in higher dimensions) using all the training data. The position of the hyperplane is determined by the support vectors—those observations closest to the boundary.

Mathematical Formulation

The decision boundary in a linear support vector machine (SVM) is defined as:

$$\mathbf{w}^{\mathrm{T}}\mathbf{x} + b = 0$$

where:

- $\mathbf{w}$ is the weight vector (containing coefficients for each feature),
- $\mathbf{x}$ is the feature vector for an observation,
- b is the bias (intercept) term.

The classification is based on the value of the decision function:

$$f(\mathbf{x}) = \mathbf{w}^{\mathrm{T}}\mathbf{x} + b$$

- If $f(\mathbf{x}) > 0$, the observation is classified into one class (e.g., "Yes" or "1").
- If $f(\mathbf{x}) \leq 0$,the observation is classified into one class (e.g., "No" or "0").

Simulated Dataset Example

To illustrate SVM, we use the simulated health dataset created previously, which contains variables such as age, gender, blood_pressure, risk (high/low), and doctors_notes. This dataset mirrors a typical public health scenario where classification is required. A useful ChatGPT prompt can be: *"Provide R code to apply a Support Vector Machine (SVM) classification on my simulated dataset, using age and blood_pressure as predictors for the risk variable. Please include code for fitting the model, predicting classes, calculating accuracy, and plotting the decision boundary."*

Based on this prompt, ChatGPT generates the example code as shown in Fig. 7.3:

r Copy Edit

```r
# Load the required package
library(e1071)

# Fit the SVM model using age and blood_pressure as predictors
svm_model <- svm(risk ~ age + blood_pressure, data = df, kernel = "linear")

# Predict on the same data (for demonstration)
pred <- predict(svm_model, df)

# Evaluate accuracy
accuracy <- mean(pred == df$risk)
print(accuracy)

# (Optional) Visualize the decision boundary if desired
library(ggplot2)
xrange <- seq(min(df$age), max(df$age), length = 100)
yrange <- seq(min(df$blood_pressure), max(df$blood_pressure), length = 100)
grid <- expand.grid(age = xrange, blood_pressure = yrange)
grid$pred <- predict(svm_model, newdata = grid)
ggplot(df, aes(x = age, y = blood_pressure, color = risk)) +
  geom_point(size = 2) +
  geom_contour(data = grid, aes(z = as.numeric(pred)), breaks = 1.5, color = "black") +
  labs(title = "SVM Decision Boundary", x = "Age", y = "Blood Pressure") +
  theme_minimal()
```

Fig. 7.3 R code generated by ChatGPT regarding how the support vector machine (SVM) algorithm is performed in RStudio

The provided R code fits a support vector machine (SVM) model to the simulated dataset in order to classify individuals as either "high" or "low" risk based on their age and blood pressure. The code then evaluates how accurately the model predicts risk and produces a visual plot showing how the SVM separates the two risk groups with a decision boundary.

Use a simple prompt such as "provide explanations of the above code" in ChatGPT, and step-by-step explanations will be provided (see Fig. 7.4):

Running the code in RStudio will generate several objects, including "df," "grid," "svm_model," and various value outputs. Most of these objects are not central to the

Explanation of the SVM Example Code

1. Load the Required Package

r Copy Edit

```r
library(e1071)
```

- **Purpose:**
  Loads the `e1071` package, which provides functions for Support Vector Machine (SVM) modeling in R.

2. Fit the SVM Model

r Copy Edit

```r
svm_model <- svm(risk ~ age + blood_pressure, data = df, kernel = "linear")
```

- **Purpose:**
  Fits an SVM classification model to the dataset `df` .
  - The target variable is `risk` (high/low).
  - Predictors are `age` and `blood_pressure` .
  - The `kernel = "linear"` argument specifies a linear boundary.

3. Predict Classes

r Copy Edit

```r
pred <- predict(svm_model, df)
```

- **Purpose:**
  Uses the trained SVM model to predict the `risk` class for each observation in the dataset.

Fig. 7.4 Explanations generated by ChatGPT regarding how the SVM algorithm is performed in RStudio

4. Evaluate Accuracy

r Copy Edit

```r
accuracy <- mean(pred == df$risk)
print(accuracy)
```

- **Purpose:**
  Calculates the classification accuracy, which is the proportion of correctly classified observations (predicted class matches actual class).
  - Prints the result as a summary performance metric.

5. Visualize the Decision Boundary (Optional)

r Copy Edit

```r
library(ggplot2)
xrange <- seq(min(df$age), max(df$age), length = 100)
yrange <- seq(min(df$blood_pressure), max(df$blood_pressure), length = 100)
grid <- expand.grid(age = xrange, blood_pressure = yrange)
grid$pred <- predict(svm_model, newdata = grid)
ggplot(df, aes(x = age, y = blood_pressure, color = risk)) +
  geom_point(size = 2) +
  geom_contour(data = grid, aes(z = as.numeric(pred)), breaks = 1.5, color = "black") +
  labs(title = "SVM Decision Boundary", x = "Age", y = "Blood Pressure") +
  theme_minimal()
```

- **Purpose:**
  - **Prepares a grid** of possible age and blood pressure values for visualization.
  - **Uses the model to predict classes** over this grid, simulating the decision surface.
  - **Creates a scatterplot** showing the actual data points colored by true `risk`.
  - **Adds a contour line** representing the SVM decision boundary (where the class assignment changes).
  - **Labels and styles the plot** for clarity.

↓

Fig. 7.4 (continued)

discussion. Of greater interest is the "accuracy" value (step 4 above), which in this example was calculated as 0.99—indicating that the model is highly accurate with the simulated data. In addition, the code produces an SVM Decision Boundary plot, as shown in Fig. 7.5:

In the plot depicted in Fig. 7.5, the SVM decision boundary is shown as the black line. This line appears on an x-y coordinate system with Age on the x-axis and Blood Pressure on the y-axis, and it separates the low- and high-risk groups. Red dots represent individuals classified as low risk, while green dots represent those classified as high risk.

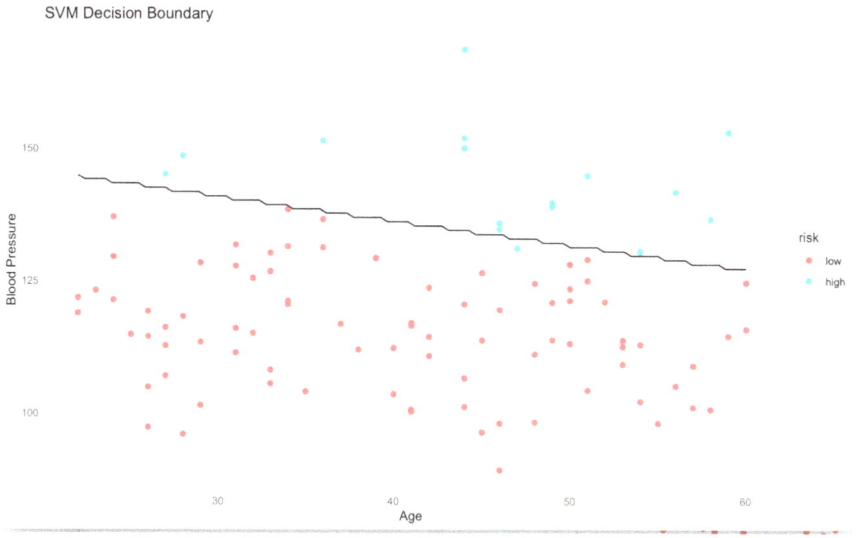

Fig. 7.5 SVM Plot produced by RStudio

Gradient Boosting (GB)

GB is a powerful supervised machine learning technique widely used for classification and prediction tasks in public health research. Unlike methods that fit a single model, GB builds an ensemble of decision trees in a sequential manner. The learning procedure consecutively fits new models to provide a more accurate estimate of the response variable (Natekin & Knoll, 2013), with each new tree trained to correct the errors made by the previous trees, resulting in a strong model that can capture complex patterns in the data.

The fundamental principle of gradient boosting lies in its iterative approach to model improvement. GB is a machine learning algorithm where multiple weak learners (tree-based classifiers) are trained to augment each other and produce superior results (Klug et al., 2020). This sequential learning process distinguishes gradient boosting from other ensemble methods like random forests, where trees are built independently. In gradient boosting, each subsequent model focuses specifically on the residual errors of the combined previous models, effectively learning from the collective mistakes to enhance overall predictive accuracy.

The algorithm's effectiveness stems from its ability to combine multiple weak learners into a single strong predictor. By iteratively adding models that target the remaining prediction errors, gradient boosting can achieve superior performance compared to individual models. This makes it particularly valuable for complex public health datasets where traditional single-model approaches may struggle to capture intricate relationships between variables such as disease risk factors, population demographics, and health outcomes. The method has demonstrated remarkable success in clinical applications, from emergency department triage systems to disease prediction models, establishing itself as a robust tool for predictive analytics in public health research.

Mathematical Formulation

The prediction from a Gradient Boosting model for a new observation x\mathbf{ x} x is expressed as the sum of outputs from many decision trees:

$$F_M(\mathbf{x}) = \sum_{m=1}^{M} \gamma_m h_m(\mathbf{x})$$

where:

- $\boldsymbol{M}$ is the total number of tres,
- $h_{\boldsymbol{m}}(\mathbf{x})$ is the prediction from the m^{th}decision tree,
- γ_m is the weight assigned to the mth tree.

  The classification is based on the value of $F_M(x)$.

- If $F_M(x) > 0$, the observation is classified into one class (e.g., "Yes" or "1").
- If $F_M(x) \leq 0$,the observation is classified into one class (e.g., "No" or "0").

Simulated Dataset Example

To illustrate Gradient Boosting, we use the same simulated health dataset with variables such as age, gender, blood_pressure, risk (high/low), and doctors_notes. This example reflects real-world scenarios where robust classification is needed. Use the ChatGPT Prompt: *"Provide R code to apply Gradient Boosting classification on my simulated dataset, using age and blood_pressure as predictors for the risk variable. Please include code for fitting the model, predicting classes, calculating accuracy, and visualizing the decision regions."* Based on this prompt, ChatGPT generates the example code as shown in Fig. 7.6:

The provided R code fits a gradient boosting model to the simulated dataset in order to classify individuals as either "high" or "low" risk based on their age and blood pressure. The code then evaluates how accurately the model predicts risk and can be extended to produce a visual plot that illustrates how gradient boosting separates the two risk groups with a flexible decision boundary. You can use a simple prompt such as "provide explanations of the above code" in ChatGPT, and step-by-step explanations will be provided for each part of the workflow (see Fig. 7.7).

r Copy Edit

```
library(xgboost)
library(ggplot2)

# Prepare label (1 = High, 0 = Low)
df$label <- ifelse(df$risk == "High", 1L, 0L)

# Fit model
xgb_data  <- xgb.DMatrix(data = as.matrix(df[, c("age", "blood_pressure")]), label = df$l
xgb_model <- xgboost(data = xgb_data, nrounds = 50, objective = "binary:logistic", verbos

# Predict on the same data
pred_prob  <- predict(xgb_model, as.matrix(df[, c("age", "blood_pressure")]))
pred_class <- factor(ifelse(pred_prob > 0.5, "High", "Low"), levels = levels(df$risk))

# Accuracy
accuracy <- mean(pred_class == df$risk)
print(paste("Accuracy:", round(accuracy, 3)))

ggplot(df, aes(x = age, y = blood_pressure, color = risk)) +
  geom_point(size = 2) +
  geom_contour(data = grid,
               aes(z = as.numeric(pred == "high")),
               breaks = 0.5,
               color = "blue") +
  labs(title = "Gradient Boosting Decision Boundary",
       x = "Age", y = "Blood Pressure") +
  theme_minimal()
```

Fig. 7.6 R code generated by ChatGPT regarding how the gradient boosting algorithm is performed in RStudio

Running the code in RStudio will generate several objects, including "df," "grid," "xgb_model," and various value outputs. Most of these objects are not central to the discussion. Of greater interest is the "accuracy" value, which in this example was calculated as 1—indicating that the gradient boosting model is perfectly accurate with the simulated data. The perfect prediction almost never happens in real data. With additional codes, we can use results from gradient boosting model to produce a decision boundary such as SVM to classify observations (e.g., high vs. low risk). The code below produces a Gradient Boosting Decision Boundary plot, as shown in Fig. 7.8:

In the plot depicted in Fig. 7.8, the Gradient Boosting Decision Boundary is shown as the blue line. This line appears on an x-y coordinate system with Age on the x-axis and Blood Pressure on the y-axis, and it separates the low- and high-risk groups. Red dots represent individuals classified as low risk, while green dots represent those classified as high risk.

1. Load libraries

- `xgboost` trains a gradient boosting (tree-based) classifier.
- `ggplot2` produces the scatter plot and (optionally) overlays a decision boundary.

2. Encode the outcome as numeric for XGBoost

r Copy Edit

```
df$label <- ifelse(df$risk == "High", 1L, 0L)
```

- Converts the categorical target `risk` into a binary label: **1 = High, 0 = Low.**
- XGBoost expects numeric labels for binary classification.

3. Build the data matrix X and label y

r Copy Edit

```
xgb_data <- xgb.DMatrix(data = as.matrix(df[, c("age", "blood_pressure")]), label = df$la
```

- Uses only two predictors, `age` and `blood_pressure`.
- Wraps them in an `xgb.DMatrix`, XGBoost's efficient data container.

4. Fit a binary logistic gradient boosting model

r Copy Edit

```
xgb_model <- xgboost(data = xgb_data, nrounds = 50, objective = "binary:logistic", verbos
```

- `objective = "binary:logistic"` trains a classifier that outputs probabilities $P(\text{High})$.
- `nrounds = 50` is the number of boosting iterations (trees).
- No hyperparameter tuning is included here; this is a quick baseline.

5. Generate predictions (probabilities) and convert to classes

r Copy Edit

```
pred_prob  <- predict(xgb_model, as.matrix(df[, c("age", "blood_pressure")]))
pred_class <- factor(ifelse(pred_prob > 0.5, "High", "Low"), levels = levels(df$risk))
```

- `predict()` returns probabilities of the **High** class.
- A 0.5 threshold converts probabilities to class labels (**High/Low**).

6. Evaluate simple accuracy

r Copy Edit

```
accuracy <- mean(pred_class == df$risk)
print(paste("Accuracy:", round(accuracy, 3)))
```

- Compares predicted vs. actual labels on the **same data used for training.**
- Useful as a quick check, but optimistic; for fair evaluation, use a train/test split or cross-validation.

Fig. 7.7 Explanations generated by ChatGPT regarding how the gradient boosting algorithm is performed in RStudio

7. Visualize points and (optionally) a decision boundary

r Copy Edit

```
ggplot(df, aes(x = age, y = blood_pressure, color = risk)) +
  geom_point(size = 2) +
  geom_contour(data = grid,
               aes(z = as.numeric(pred == "high")),
               breaks = 0.5,
               color = "blue") +
  labs(title = "Gradient Boosting Decision Boundary",
       x = "Age", y = "Blood Pressure") +
  theme_minimal()
```

- The scatter shows observed cases colored by **actual** risk.
- The contour intends to draw the **decision boundary** where the model flips classes (around probability 0.5).
- **Important prerequisite:** this contour layer assumes you have a `grid` data frame with columns `age`, `blood_pressure`, and a `pred` vector of predicted classes (e.g., `"high"` / `"low"`) computed over a mesh of points. If `grid` / `pred` don't exist, add a grid-generation step and predict on it before plotting.

Fig. 7.7 (continued)

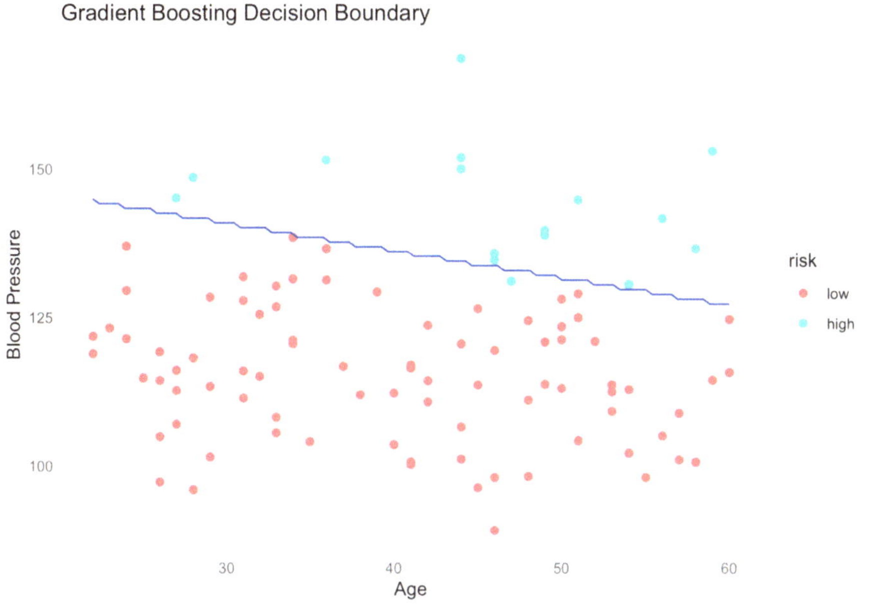

Fig. 7.8 Gradient Boosting Decision Boundary graph produced by RStudio

Deep Learning (DL)

DL is an advanced machine learning technique increasingly applied in public health for complex classification and prediction tasks. It utilizes computational models with multiple processing layers ("deep" architectures) to learn data representations with multiple levels of abstraction and extract intricate patterns from large datasets (LeCun et al., 2015). Compared with traditional models or ensemble methods, DL is more effective at capturing non-linear relationships and subtle interactions among predictors. This capability makes DL a powerful tool for analyzing high-dimensional data, where conventional models may fall short.

The fundamental principle of deep learning lies in its hierarchical structure. A deep neural network consists of an input layer (for predictors), one or more hidden layers (which transform and combine inputs), and an output layer (for the predicted class or value). Each layer is made up of interconnected nodes, called neurons, which apply mathematical transformations and non-linear activation functions. Through iterative training, the network adjusts its internal weights to minimize prediction errors, learning increasingly abstract representations of the data at each layer.

This multi-layered learning process distinguishes deep learning from other machine learning techniques. While methods like gradient boosting rely on sequentially combining weak learners, deep learning learns complex representations directly from the data, enabling superior performance on high-dimensional and unstructured datasets such as electronic health records, imaging data, or free-text clinical notes. Deep learning has demonstrated remarkable success in various health and management applications, from disease risk prediction to image-based diagnostics and natural language processing (Esteva et al., 2019).

Mathematical Formulation

The prediction from a deep neural network for an observation x\mathbf{ x}x can be expressed as a series of transformations through multiple layers:

$$\mathbf{h}^{(l)} = \boldsymbol{f}^{(l)}\left(\mathbf{W}^{(l)}\mathbf{h}^{(l-1)} + \mathbf{b}^{(l)}\right), \qquad \boldsymbol{l} = \mathbf{1}, \mathbf{2}, \ldots, \boldsymbol{L}$$

where:

- $\mathbf{h}^{(l)}$ is the output of the l^{th}layer (with $\mathbf{h}^{(0)} = \mathrm{x}$)
- $f^{(l)}$ is the activation function for the l^{th}layer,
- $\mathbf{W}^{(l)}$ and $b^{(l)}$ are the weights and biases for the lth layer,
- L is the total number of layers.

The final output layer generates the class prediction (e.g., high or low risk) by applying a suitable activation function (e.g., softmax or sigmoid).

Simulated Dataset Example

To illustrate deep learning, we use the same simulated health dataset with variables such as age, gender, blood_pressure, risk (high/low), and doctors_notes. This example reflects real-world management and public health scenarios where advanced classification is needed.

We will use this prompt in ChatGPT: "Provide R code to apply a deep learning (neural network) model to my simulated dataset, using age and blood_pressure as predictors for the risk variable. Please include code for fitting the model, predicting classes, calculating accuracy, and visualizing the decision regions." Based on this prompt, ChatGPT generates the example code as shown in Fig. 7.9:

The provided R code fits a deep learning (neural network) model to the simulated dataset in order to classify individuals as either "high" or "low" risk based on their age and blood pressure. The code then evaluates the model's predictive accuracy and produces a visual plot illustrating how deep learning separates the two risk groups with a flexible and potentially non-linear decision boundary. You can use a simple prompt such as "provide explanations of the above code on deep learning" in ChatGPT to receive detailed, step-by-step explanations of each part of the workflow (see Fig. 7.10).

Running the code in RStudio will generate several objects, including "df," "grid," "nn_model," and various value outputs. Most of these objects are not central to the discussion. Of greater interest is the "accuracy" value, which in this example was calculated as 0.83—indicating that the deep learning model achieves a high level of predictive accuracy with the simulated data. It should be noted that such performance is typical for moderately complex datasets, as perfect prediction is rarely achieved in real-world applications. With additional code, we can use the results from the deep learning model to produce a decision boundary plot, similar to those created for SVM or gradient boosting, to classify observations (e.g., high vs. low risk). The code below produces a Deep Learning Decision Boundary plot, as shown in Fig. 7.11:

In the plot depicted in Fig. 7.11, the Deep Learning decision boundary is shown as the purple line. This line appears on an x-y coordinate system with Age on the x-axis and Blood Pressure on the y-axis, and it separates the low- and high-risk groups. Red dots represent individuals classified as low risk, while green dots represent those classified as high risk.

Natural Language Processing (NLP)

Natural Language Processing (NLP) is a specialized area of machine learning focused on analyzing and extracting meaningful information from unstructured text data. In management and public health research, NLP methods are increasingly used to process clinical notes, patient comments, or other free-text sources to support

r Copy Edit

```r
# 1) Neural network (nnet) — binary classification for risk
library(nnet)

# Prepare binary label: 1 = High, 0 = Low
df$label <- ifelse(df$risk == "High", 1, 0)

# 2) Fit model (2 inputs -> hidden size 4 -> 1 output)
nn_model <- nnet(label ~ age + blood_pressure,
                 data = df,
                 size = 4, maxit = 500, trace = FALSE)

# 3) Predict probabilities and classes
nn_pred_prob <- as.numeric(predict(nn_model, df, type = "raw"))
nn_pred <- ifelse(nn_pred_prob > 0.5, "High", "Low")

# 4) Accuracy
accuracy <- mean(nn_pred == df$risk)
print(paste("Accuracy:", round(accuracy, 3)))

# 5) Visualization of decision regions
library(ggplot2)

xrange <- seq(min(df$age, na.rm = TRUE), max(df$age, na.rm = TRUE), length.out = 200)
yrange <- seq(min(df$blood_pressure, na.rm = TRUE), max(df$blood_pressure, na.rm = TRUE),
grid <- expand.grid(age = xrange, blood_pressure = yrange)

grid$pred_prob <- as.numeric(predict(nn_model, grid, type = "raw"))

ggplot(df, aes(x = age, y = blood_pressure, color = risk)) +
  geom_point(size = 2) +
  geom_contour(data = grid,
               aes(x = age, y = blood_pressure, z = pred_prob),
               breaks = 0.5, color = "black") +
  labs(title = "Neural Network Decision Boundary",
       x = "Age", y = "Blood Pressure") +
  theme_minimal()
```

Fig. 7.9 R code generated by ChatGPT regarding how the deep learning algorithm is performed in RStudio

classification, prediction, and decision-making (Sheikhalishahi et al., 2019). Unlike traditional models that rely on structured numeric or categorical data, NLP enables researchers to leverage qualitative variables, such as doctors' notes, for more comprehensive and nuanced analyses.

The fundamental principle of NLP in predictive analytics is the transformation of raw text into structured features that can be incorporated into statistical or machine learning models. Common approaches include generating binary indicators (e.g.,

1) Load the package

- `library(nnet)` : enables a **single-hidden-layer neural network** for classification/regression.

2) Create the binary target

- `df$label <- ifelse(df$risk == "High", 1, 0)` : converts the categorical **risk** into a numeric label (1 = High, 0 = Low) required by `nnet()` for classification.

3) Fit the neural network

- `nnet_model <- nnet(label ~ age + blood_pressure, data = df, size = 4, maxit = 500, trace = FALSE)`
  - **Formula**: predict `label` from `age` and `blood_pressure`.
  - **size = 4**: four hidden units (nonlinear capacity).
  - **maxit = 500**: maximum optimization iterations.
  - **trace = FALSE**: suppresses training output.
  - Practical note: neural nets are sensitive to scaling; standardizing predictors often improves stability/performance.

4) Predict and classify

- `nn_pred_prob <- as.numeric(predict(nn_model, df, type = "raw"))` : predicted **probability of High** for each case.
- `nn_pred <- ifelse(nn_pred_prob > 0.5, "High", "Low")` : converts probabilities to classes using a 0.5 threshold (adjust if you need higher sensitivity/specificity).

5) Evaluate accuracy

- `accuracy <- mean(nn_pred == df$risk)` : share of correct classifications on the same data used to train (a **quick but optimistic** check).
- For decision quality, prefer a train/test split or cross-validation.

6) Visualize decision regions

- `xrange`, `yrange` : create evenly spaced sequences across the ranges of **age** and **blood_pressure**.
- `grid <- expand.grid(...)` : forms a mesh of points over the feature space.
- `grid$pred_prob <- predict(nn_model, grid, type = "raw")` : computes the model's probability at each grid point.
- `ggplot(...)+ geom_point(...)` : plots the observed cases colored by actual **risk**.
- `geom_contour(..., z = pred_prob, breaks = 0.5)` : draws the **decision boundary** (the curve where predicted probability = 0.5).
  - Interpretation: points on one side are classified "High," the other "Low," revealing how the NN partitions the space.

Fig. 7.10 Explanations generated by ChatGPT regarding how the decision tree algorithm is performed in RStudio

whether a keyword appears in a note), counting word frequencies, or creating more advanced representations such as term frequency-inverse document frequency (TF-IDF) or word embeddings (Harrison & Sidey-Gibbons, 2021). These features can then be used to enhance the predictive power of models for tasks such as disease risk classification, symptom monitoring, or resource allocation.

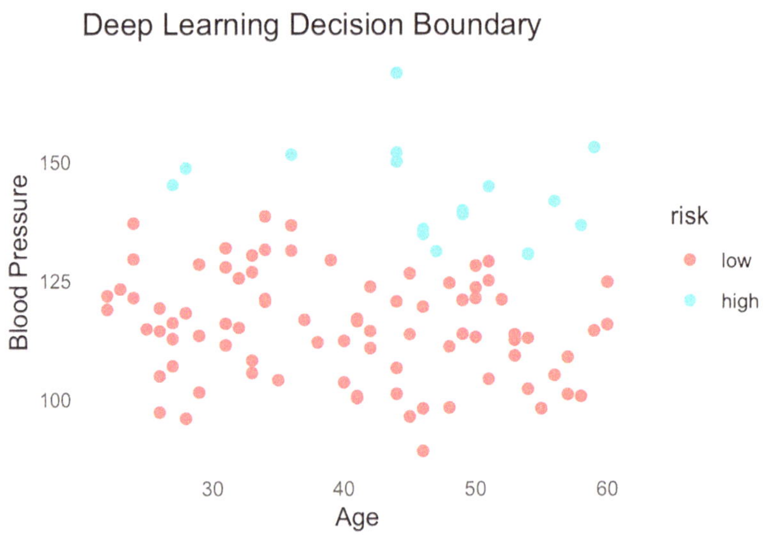

Fig. 7.11 Deep learning decision boundary

In practice, NLP augments existing modeling techniques by extracting and quantifying qualitative information that may be correlated with outcomes of interest. For example, in clinical or operational management settings, automated text analysis of medical records can identify patterns or keywords associated with high-risk cases, thus supporting timely intervention and improved decision-making.

Simulated Dataset Example

To illustrate NLP, we use the same simulated health dataset, which includes age, gender, blood_pressure, risk (high/low), and doctors_notes. Here, the doctors_notes variable provides unstructured clinical notes that can be explored using NLP techniques to summarize key themes and frequently mentioned terms, rather than for predictive modeling. We use the prompt: "Provide R code to preprocess and summarize the text in the doctors_notes variable in my simulated dataset, including steps for cleaning the text, identifying the most common words, and visualizing the results with a word cloud." Based on this prompt, ChatGPT generates the example code as shown in Fig. 7.12:

The provided R code demonstrates how NLP methods can be applied to extract features from clinical notes (for example, detecting mention of "pain") and include them in a predictive model. The resulting model classifies individuals as either "high" or "low" risk based on both traditional predictors and text-derived features, and the code evaluates the model's accuracy. Visualization of the decision boundary further illustrates the potential impact of incorporating qualitative text data into risk

r Copy Edit

```r
# Install required packages if not already installed
if (!require("tm")) install.packages("tm")
if (!require("wordcloud")) install.packages("wordcloud")
if (!require("RColorBrewer")) install.packages("RColorBrewer")

library(tm)
library(wordcloud)
library(RColorBrewer)

# Assume your data frame is named df and contains the 'doctors_notes' variable

# Step 1: Create a text corpus
corpus <- Corpus(VectorSource(df$doctors_notes))

# Step 2: Clean the text
corpus <- tm_map(corpus, content_transformer(tolower))          # Convert to lowerca
corpus <- tm_map(corpus, removePunctuation)                      # Remove punctuation
corpus <- tm_map(corpus, removeNumbers)                          # Remove numbers (if
corpus <- tm_map(corpus, removeWords, stopwords("en"))           # Remove common stop
corpus <- tm_map(corpus, stripWhitespace)                        # Remove extra white

# Step 2: Clean the text
corpus <- tm_map(corpus, content_transformer(tolower))          # Convert to lowerca
corpus <- tm_map(corpus, removePunctuation)                      # Remove punctuation
corpus <- tm_map(corpus, removeNumbers)                          # Remove numbers (if
corpus <- tm_map(corpus, removeWords, stopwords("en"))           # Remove common stop
corpus <- tm_map(corpus, stripWhitespace)                        # Remove extra white

# Step 3: Create a document-term matrix
dtm <- TermDocumentMatrix(corpus)
m <- as.matrix(dtm)

# Step 4: Calculate word frequencies
word_freqs <- sort(rowSums(m), decreasing = TRUE)

# Step 5: Display the top 10 most common words
print(head(word_freqs, 10))

# Step 6: Visualize with a word cloud
set.seed(123) # For reproducibility
wordcloud(words = names(word_freqs),
          freq = word_freqs,
          min.freq = 1,
          scale = c(3, 0.5),
          colors = brewer.pal(8, "Dark2"),
          random.order = FALSE)
```

Fig. 7.12 R code generated by ChatGPT regarding how natural language processing (NLP) algorithm is performed in RStudio

classification. You can use a simple prompt such as "provide explanations of the above code on nlp" in ChatGPT to receive detailed, step-by-step explanations of each part of the workflow (see Fig. 7.13).

Running the code in RStudio will generate several objects, including "df," "corpus," "dtm," and various value outputs. Most of these objects are not central to the discussion. Of greater interest are the word frequencies and the word cloud produced above, which visually summarize the most common terms found in the doctors' notes. This analysis highlights recurring themes and key language patterns in the qualitative clinical data. In Step 7, a word cloud was created. The word cloud provides an intuitive overview of which words are most prominent in the dataset, as shown in Fig. 7.14:

Users may also use "print(head(word_freqs, 10))" in RStudio to inspect the top 10 most common words in RStudio for the "doctors_notes" variable in the simulated dataset (see Fig. 7.15):

Comparison of Advanced Machine Learning Models

Advanced machine learning models discussed in this chapter—including Support Vector Machine (SVM), gradient boosting, deep learning, and Natural Language Processing (NLP) approaches—are important tools for classification, prediction, and pattern recognition in public health research. These models vary in methodology, interpretability, flexibility, and suitability for different types of data and research objectives (Kather et al., 2019).

Table 7.1 summarizes key similarities and differences among these four foundational approaches, highlighting their typical use cases and best practices with the simulated health dataset.

Summary

All four approaches are designed to extract meaningful insights from complex data, supporting decision-making and strategy in public health. SVM, gradient boosting, and deep learning are primarily supervised learning models requiring labeled outcome variables and are widely used for classification and prediction (Rashidi et al., 2023). NLP, while not a classifier itself, transforms unstructured text into features that can be summarized descriptively or included in predictive models (Jerfy et al., 2024).

However, these models vary in their relative strengths, computational requirements, and levels of interpretability and flexibility.

SVM algorithms are particularly effective in defining decision boundaries that distinguish patient groups based on their risk profiles. This makes them well-suited for public and population health applications. By incorporating genomic,

Explanation of the NLP Code for Summarizing Doctors' Notes

1. Install and Load Required Packages

r Copy Edit

```r
if (!require("tm")) install.packages("tm")
if (!require("wordcloud")) install.packages("wordcloud")
if (!require("RColorBrewer")) install.packages("RColorBrewer")
library(tm)
library(wordcloud)
library(RColorBrewer)
```

- **Purpose:**
  Ensures the necessary packages (`tm` for text mining, `wordcloud` for visualization, `RColorBrewer` for color palettes) are installed and loaded into your R session.

2. Create a Text Corpus

r Copy Edit

```r
corpus <- Corpus(VectorSource(df$doctors_notes))
```

- **Purpose:**
  Converts the `doctors_notes` column from your data frame into a **corpus**, which is a standard format for handling collections of text documents in NLP.

3. Clean and Preprocess the Text

r Copy Edit

```r
corpus <- tm_map(corpus, content_transformer(tolower))      # Convert all text to low
corpus <- tm_map(corpus, removePunctuation)                 # Remove punctuation mark
corpus <- tm_map(corpus, removeNumbers)                     # Remove any numbers (if
corpus <- tm_map(corpus, removeWords, stopwords("en"))      # Remove common English s
corpus <- tm_map(corpus, stripWhitespace)                   # Eliminate extra spaces
```

- **Purpose:**
  These steps standardize the text and remove irrelevant elements, ensuring that the analysis focuses on meaningful words only.

Fig. 7.13 Explanations generated by ChatGPT regarding how natural language processing (NLP) is performed in RStudio

4. Create a Document-Term Matrix

r Copy Edit

```r
dtm <- TermDocumentMatrix(corpus)
m <- as.matrix(dtm)
```

- **Purpose:**
  Builds a matrix where each row represents a unique word, each column represents a document (doctor's note), and each entry is the frequency of that word in the document. This matrix enables efficient analysis of word frequencies.

5. Calculate Word Frequencies

r Copy Edit

```r
word_freqs <- sort(rowSums(m), decreasing = TRUE)
```

- **Purpose:**
  Sums the frequency of each word across all documents, sorts them in descending order, and creates a list of the most frequently mentioned terms in the clinical notes.

6. Display the Top 10 Most Common Words

r Copy Edit

```r
print(head(word_freqs, 10))
```

- **Purpose:**
  Outputs the ten most commonly used words in the doctors' notes. This helps reveal recurring themes or concerns documented by clinicians.

Fig. 7.13 (continued)

demographic, and clinical variables, SVM can classify patients according to their likelihood of developing certain diseases (Uddin et al., 2024). Such applications are especially valuable for identifying high-risk cohorts who may benefit from targeted preventive interventions, such as diabetes management programs or cardiac rehabilitation.

GB methods have become widely recognized for their strong predictive power in clinical decision support. Through their ensemble approach—sequentially

7. Visualize Results with a Word Cloud

r

Copy Edit

```r
set.seed(123) # For reproducibility
wordcloud(words = names(word_freqs),
          freq = word_freqs,
          min.freq = 1,
          scale = c(3, 0.5),
          colors = brewer.pal(8, "Dark2"),
          random.order = FALSE)
```

- **Purpose:**
  Creates a word cloud, where more frequent words appear larger and bolder. This visualization provides a quick, intuitive summary of the most prominent topics and themes in the qualitative notes.

Fig. 7.13 (continued)

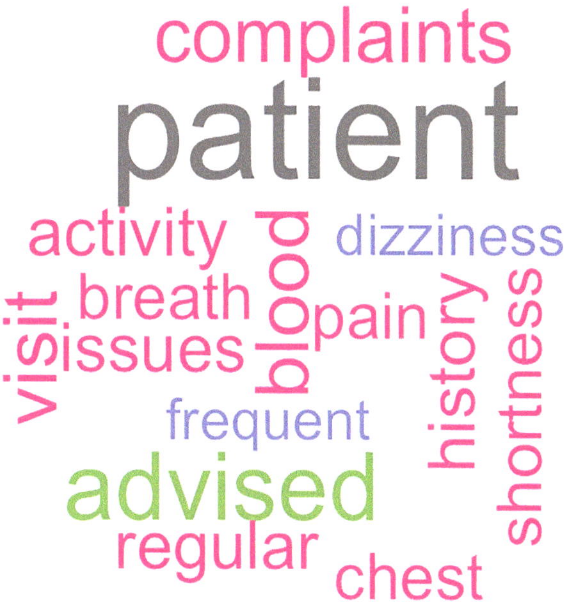

Fig. 7.14 A word cloud using the corpus of "doctors_notes" variable in the simulated dataset created in RStudio

combining weak learners to build robust predictors—these models have shown high accuracy in contexts such as emergency department triage, where they help identify patients at heightened risk of early mortality (Raita et al., 2019). Clinicians also appreciate their ability to highlight variable importance, offering transparency into which clinical factors most strongly shape outcomes.

```
> print(head(word_freqs, 10))
   patient     reports     advised      intake      reduce
        37          26          23          23          23
      salt     checkup  complaints     routine significant
        23          18          18          18          18
>
```

Fig. 7.15 The top 10 keywords from the corpus of "doctors_notes" variable in the simulated dataset

Table 7.1 Comparison of 4 advanced ML models: Support Vector Machine (SVM), Gradient Boosting (GB), Deep Learning (DL), and Natural Language Processing (NLP)

Model	Key features	Typical use/purpose	Illustrative dataset	Similarities	Differences
SVM	Maximizes margin; linear/ non-linear boundaries	Binary/ multiclass classification; risk prediction	Simulated health data (focus on classification)	Supervised, uses labeled data, needs feature selection	Provides interpretable boundaries; limited with large/complex data
GB	Ensemble of decision trees; sequential error correction	High-accuracy prediction; non-linear classification	Simulated health data (focus on classification)	Supervised, robust to overfitting, flexible	Less interpretable; requires careful tuning
DL	Multi-layer neural networks; automatic feature learning	Complex, non-linear pattern recognition; image/text	Simulated health data (focus on classification)	Supervised, handles large/ unstructured data	Requires large datasets; less transparent ("black box")
NLP	Text feature extraction; pattern mining from unstructured text	Theme detection, summarization, qualitative insights	Simulated health data (focus on doctors' notes)	Can enhance other models, enables qualitative analysis	Not predictive by itself; best for text exploration or feature engineering

DL and related neural networks frameworks have advanced public health research by enabling the analysis of complex, multimodal data sources, including medical imaging, laboratory test results, and clinical documentation. Combining natural language processing with image analysis provides complementary insights, improving both diagnostic accuracy and patient care (Vellido et al., 2024). Notable applications include automated detection of diabetic retinopathy, identification of skin cancer, and prediction of patient deterioration using continuous monitoring data integrated with electronic health records.

NLP is increasingly important for clinical intelligence, as much of medical information exists in unstructured text such as physician notes and nursing documentation. Leveraging NLP with machine learning makes it possible to extract actionable insights, improve diagnostic accuracy, and enhance surveillance of care quality and patient safety (Vellido et al., 2024). Applied to electronic health records and imaging systems, NLP allows healthcare organizations to perform automated, near real-time monitoring of clinical narratives for better decision-making.

Modern healthcare systems increasingly deploy these ML approaches in combination, leveraging each method's strengths for comprehensive patient care. The integration of these ML methods has transformed healthcare from reactive treatment models to proactive, predictive care systems that can identify at-risk populations before symptoms appear and continuously monitor care quality through automated analysis.

Discussion Questions

1. How can supervised learning models like SVM, gradient boosting, or deep learning support decision-making in public health?
2. What are the primary trade-offs between model interpretability and predictive performance when selecting among SVM, gradient boosting, and deep learning?
3. In what ways can NLP be integrated with structured data analysis to enrich public health research?
4. What strategies can be used to assess and compare the real-world impact of these advanced models in applied public health settings?
5. What ethical and governance issues arise when applying these models to sensitive health data?

References

Beam, A. L., & Kohane, I. S. (2018). Big data and machine learning in health care. *JAMA, 319*(13), 1317–1318. https://doi.org/10.1001/jama.2017.18391

Chen, J. H., & Asch, S. M. (2017). Machine learning and prediction in medicine—Beyond the peak of inflated expectations. *New England Journal of Medicine, 376*(26), 2507–2509. https://doi.org/10.1056/NEJMp1702071

Esteva, A., Robicquet, A., Ramsundar, B., Kuleshov, V., DePristo, M., Chou, K., Cui, C., Corrado, G., Thrun, S., & Dean, J. (2019). A guide to deep learning in healthcare. *Nature Medicine, 25*(1), 24–29. https://doi.org/10.1038/s41591-018-0316-z

Harrison, C. J., & Sidey-Gibbons, C. J. (2021). Machine learning in medicine: A practical introduction to natural language processing. *BMC Medical Research Methodology, 21*, 158. https://doi.org/10.1186/s12874-021-01347-1

Huang, S., Cai, N., Pacheco, P. P., Narrandes, S., Wang, Y., & Xu, W. (2018). Applications of support vector machine (SVM) learning in cancer genomics. *Cancer Genomics & Proteomics, 15*(1), 41–51. https://doi.org/10.21873/cgp.20063

James, G., Witten, D., Hastie, T., & Tibshirani, R. (2021). *An introduction to statistical learning: With applications in R* (2nd ed.). Springer. https://www.statlearning.com/

Jerfy, A., Selden, O., & Balkrishnan, R. (2024). The growing impact of natural language processing in healthcare and public health. *Inquiry, 61*, 469580241290095. https://doi.org/10.1177/00469580241290095

Kasneci, E., Seßler, K., Küchemann, S., Bannert, M., Dementieva, D., Fischer, F., Gasser, U., Groh, G., Günnemann, S., Hüllermeier, E., Krusche, S., Kutyniok, G., Michaeli, T., Nerdel, C., Pfeffer, J., Poquet, O., Sailer, M., Schmidt, A., Seidel, T., et al. (2023). ChatGPT for good?

On opportunities and challenges of large language models for education. *Learning and Individual Differences, 103*, 102274. https://doi.org/10.1016/j.lindif.2023.102274

Kather, J. N., Pearson, A. T., Halama, N., Jäger, D., Krause, J., Loosen, S. H., Marx, A., Boor, P., Tacke, F., Neumann, U. P., Grabsch, H. I., Yoshikawa, T., Brenner, H., Chang-Claude, J., Hoffmeister, M., Trautwein, C., & Luedde, T. (2019). Deep learning can predict microsatellite instability directly from histology in gastrointestinal cancer. *Nature Medicine, 25*(7), 1054–1056. https://doi.org/10.1038/s41591-019-0462-y

Klug, M., Barash, Y., Bechler, S., Resheff, Y. S., Tron, T., Ironi, A., Soffer, S., Zimlichman, E., & Klang, E. (2020). A gradient boosting machine learning model for predicting early mortality in the emergency department triage: Devising a nine-point triage score. *Journal of General Internal Medicine, 35*(1), 220–227. https://doi.org/10.1007/s11606-019-05512-7

LeCun, Y., Bengio, Y., & Hinton, G. (2015). Deep learning. *Nature, 521*(7553), 436–444. https://doi.org/10.1038/nature14539

Natekin, A., & Knoll, A. (2013). Gradient boosting machines, a tutorial. *Frontiers in Neurorobotics, 7*, 21. https://pmc.ncbi.nlm.nih.gov/articles/PMC3885826/

Raita, Y., Goto, T., Faridi, M. K., Brown, D. F., Camargo, C. A., Jr., & Hasegawa, K. (2019). Emergency department triage prediction of clinical outcomes using machine learning models. *Critical Care, 23*(1), 64. https://pmc.ncbi.nlm.nih.gov/articles/PMC6957629/

Rajkomar, A., Dean, J., & Kohane, I. (2019). Machine learning in medicine. *New England Journal of Medicine, 380*(14), 1347–1359. https://doi.org/10.1056/NEJMra1814259

Rashidi, H. H., Albahra, S., Robertson, S., Tran, N. K., & Hu, B. (2023). Common statistical concepts in the supervised Machine Learning arena. *Frontiers in Oncology, 13*, 1130229. https://www.frontiersin.org/journals/oncology/articles/10.3389/fonc.2023.1130229/full

Rodríguez-Pérez, R., & Bajorath, J. (2022). Evolution of support vector machine and regression modeling in chemoinformatics and drug discovery. *Journal of Computer-Aided Molecular Design, 36*(5), 355–362. https://doi.org/10.1007/s10822-022-00442-9

Sheikhalishahi, S., Miotto, R., Dudley, J. T., Lavelli, A., Rinaldi, F., & Osmani, V. (2019). Natural language processing of clinical notes on chronic diseases: Systematic review. *JMIR Medical Informatics, 7*(2), e12239. https://doi.org/10.2196/12239

Uddin, S., Khan, A., Hossain, M. E., & Moni, M. A. (2024). An overview on the advancements of support vector machine models in healthcare applications: A review. *Information, 15*(4), 235. https://www.mdpi.com/2078-2489/15/4/235

Vellido, A., Ribas, V., Morales, C., Sanmartín, A., & Minguillón, J. (2024). Advancements and gaps in natural language processing and machine learning applications in healthcare: A comprehensive review of electronic medical records and medical imaging. *Frontiers in Physics, 12*, 1445204. https://www.frontiersin.org/journals/physics/articles/10.3389/fphy.2024.1445204/full

Part III
Ethical, Responsible, and Real-World AI Applications

Chapter 8
Real-World Applications of Supervised Learning

Learning Objectives
By the end of this chapter, readers will be able to:

1. **Apply** advanced supervised learning algorithms to classify health outcomes using EHR data.
2. **Compare** logistic regression, decision tree, and random forest classifiers in RStudio.
3. **Evaluate** classification model performance using comprehensive metrics including accuracy, sensitivity, specificity, and ROC curves.
4. **Interpret** advanced model outputs to inform public health decision-making and policy development.
5. **Leverage** generative AI tools strategically to enhance coding efficiency, model interpretation, and troubleshooting in supervised learning workflows.

Real-World Application Using Simulated Electronic Health Record Data (EHR)

Building upon the foundations of supervised learning introduced in Chap. 4, this chapter explores the application of classification techniques using simulated electronic health record (EHR) data. The primary aim is to demonstrate how machine learning (ML) can be applied to address real-world public health challenges through predictive modeling and decision support. In doing so, we introduce evaluation metrics that are essential for comparing model performance in practical contexts.

As an introductory text, we focus on classification models due to their relative interpretability and ease of use—key features for clinical decision-making. By

---

Supplementary Information The online version contains supplementary material available at https://doi.org/10.1007/978-3-032-08677-8_8.

R. Leung, *Leveraging GenAI for Machine Learning Education in Public Health*,
https://doi.org/10.1007/978-3-032-08677-8_8

applying these models to simulated EHR data, we provide readers with a hands-on understanding of ML methods and prepare them for more advanced applications, such as unsupervised learning, deep learning, and natural language processing, which may be addressed in future volumes (Chen & Asch, 2017).

The simulated dataset includes realistic clinical and behavioral variables commonly found in actual EHR systems. Through this case study, we illustrate the transformative potential of ML in healthcare delivery. When properly implemented, ML tools can assist clinicians in risk stratification and early intervention, offering a proactive approach to managing population health. For example, predictive algorithms can identify individuals at high risk of disease before symptoms manifest, enabling more timely and targeted interventions (Rajkomar et al., 2019). This capacity not only improves individual health outcomes but may also reduce the overall burden on healthcare systems.

Our case example centers on predicting substance use disorder (SUD), a persistent and globally significant public health issue. In the USA, SUD presents complex challenges, with wide disparities in incidence and treatment outcomes across populations and regions (Mokdad et al., 2018). This case study illustrates how ML can uncover hidden patterns in health data, offering insights that can inform both clinical care and public health strategy—particularly in ways that traditional methods may overlook.

At the same time, this example reveals practical challenges in applying ML to health informatics. For instance, while random forest models often outperform logistic regression and decision trees on several performance metrics—especially when modeling non-linear relationships (Goldstein et al., 2017)—they do so at the expense of transparency. This reduced explainability may limit their clinical adoption, where interpretability is essential for building provider trust and facilitating patient engagement.

The key question, then, is: how should practitioners choose the most appropriate model for a given clinical or public health application? In the following sections, we provide a framework for understanding model performance, interpretability, and implementation trade-offs to support informed decision-making in health-related ML applications.

Dataset Description

The simulated EHR dataset used in this chapter mirrors essential characteristics typically found in public health data systems. As the backbone of contemporary healthcare delivery, electronic health records incorporate both structured and unstructured information that can support predictive modeling, clinical decision-making, and population health management (Menachemi & Collum, 2011). The widespread implementation of EHRs—accelerated by federal incentive programs—has expanded opportunities for applying machine learning to improve patient outcomes while managing healthcare costs (Adler-Milstein et al., 2017). Beyond clinical care, EHR systems help organizations develop dynamic capabilities for data-driven decision-making and continuous improvement (Leung, 2012).

The dataset integrates demographic, clinical, behavioral, and psychosocial variables relevant to risk prediction and classification for substance use disorder (SUD). It serves as the core data resource for Chaps. 8 and 9. The dataset can be downloaded here: https://livememphis-my.sharepoint.com/my?id=%2Fpersonal%2Frcleung%5Fmemphis%5Fedu%2FDocuments%2FGenAI%20Book%20Datasets&ga=1

Variables

Demographic variables include *age* (a continuous variable), *gender* (a categorical variable with male and female categories), and *income level* (an ordinal variable with low, medium, and high categories). These variables reflect key social determinants of health, which strongly influence both treatment access and exposure to risk conditions associated with substance use disorders.

Clinical indicators constitute the physiological measurements commonly recorded in EHRs. *Body mass index (BMI)* is included as a continuous variable representing a key anthropometric measure. *Systolic* and *diastolic blood pressure* are each treated as continuous variables, offering insight into cardiovascular health. Similarly, *cholesterol* and *glucose* levels are included as continuous variables, reflecting critical biomarkers of metabolic health and comorbidities frequently associated with SUD.

Behavioral variables capture modifiable lifestyle factors that significantly affect health outcomes. *Smoking status* is a categorical variable with three levels: never, former, and current smokers. *Exercise frequency* is coded as an ordinal variable with low, moderate, and high levels of physical activity. These behaviors often co-occur with substance use and provide important context for understanding health risks.

Mental health status is represented by a *mental health score* ranging from 0 to 100, with higher scores indicating better psychological well-being. This continuous variable is critical for assessing treatment engagement, relapse potential, and coordination of care. *Family history of substance use* is included as a binary variable (0 = no family history; 1 = presence of family history), reflecting genetic and environmental risk factors that contribute to vulnerability and inform targeted prevention strategies.

SUD_Status serves as the primary classification outcome, coded as a binary variable (0 = no SUD; 1 = presence of SUD). This outcome represents a meaningful and realistic challenge for classification modeling in health analytics, with broad implications for public health and clinical management.

Finally, *hospital visits* is included as a continuous variable to reflect recent inpatient healthcare utilization. Although not a primary outcome in the classification model, this variable provides additional utility for future regression analysis and cost evaluation and supports broader assessments of system-level care burden.

Data Generation and Access

To support hands-on learning, the simulated dataset used in this book is available for download on the companion website. All examples in this section—and in subsequent chapters—draw directly from this dataset to ensure consistency and reproducibility. For readers interested in generating their own simulated data, ChatGPT can be a useful tool when guided by a well-structured prompt. For example, the following prompt can be used to create a similar dataset:

> Generate a realistic simulated EHR dataset with demographic, clinical, behavioral, and mental health variables for 1000 patients, including a binary outcome related to substance use disorder. Use the set.seed command to ensure reproducibility. Save the data in CSV format.

This prompt instructs ChatGPT to generate a structured dataset and output it in CSV format. Once created, the file can be downloaded to a local computer and imported into RStudio using the `read.csv()` function for further analysis. It is important to note that because ChatGPT is a large language model (LLM), the data it produces are probabilistic rather than deterministic. As OpenAI notes, "*Outputs may vary depending on the phrasing of the prompt or other stochastic factors in the generation process.*" Therefore, a dataset generated using the example prompt above will not exactly match the one used in this book, even if the instructions appear the same.

To maintain consistency across chapters and ensure replicable examples, readers are encouraged to use the dataset provided on the book's companion website.

Imaginary Case Scenario: Public Health Agency Initiative on Substance Use Disorder Using Simulated EHR Data

To contextualize the dataset and illustrate its practical relevance, consider an imaginary initiative launched by a regional public health agency to address the growing crisis of substance use disorder (SUD). In response to a surge in opioid-related overdoses and the increasing prevalence of co-occurring mental health conditions, the agency convened a cross-sector coalition comprising local hospitals, behavioral health clinics, and social service organizations. The coalition's goal is to leverage data-driven decision-making to identify risk factors and support early intervention strategies.

As part of its analytic infrastructure, the agency developed a de-identified EHR dataset to build predictive models that inform both clinical and public health responses. The simulated dataset featured in this book mirrors this hypothetical use case, consisting of 1000 individuals and capturing a wide range of demographic, clinical, behavioral, and psychosocial variables. It is designed to support three key objectives:

1. Identifying individuals at elevated risk of relapse or hospitalization,
2. Targeting preventive and behavioral interventions, and.
3. Evaluating service utilization and health outcomes across diverse population groups.

This case scenario is carried throughout Sect. "Imaginary Case Scenario: Public Health Agency Initiative on Substance Use Disorder Using Simulated EHR Data" to demonstrate the application of classification, regression, and machine learning techniques in a structured and realistic setting. It exemplifies how public health agencies and researchers might organize and analyze real-world EHR data to inform strategic planning. By simulating a practical response to SUD, the scenario highlights how machine learning can be responsibly applied to enhance treatment planning, optimize resource allocation, and strengthen population health management.

Data Preparation in RStudio

Building on the imaginary case scenario and the structure of the simulated EHR dataset, this section introduces advanced data preparation techniques essential for implementing machine learning models in the context of substance use disorder (SUD) prediction. As discussed in earlier chapters, raw data often require cleaning and preprocessing before they can be effectively used for modeling. Here, we expand on that foundation to address the specific challenges associated with preparing complex health data for classification tasks.

Electronic health records typically contain a mix of variable types, including categorical variables (e.g., *gender*, *income level*, *smoking status*), ordinal variables (e.g., *exercise frequency*), binary variables (e.g., *family history*, *SUD_Status*), and continuous variables (e.g., *age*, *BMI*, *blood pressure*, *cholesterol*, *glucose*, *mental health score*, *hospital visits*). In their raw form, these variables may not be suitable for direct use in machine learning algorithms. Preprocessing is therefore a critical step to improve model accuracy, interpretability, and computational efficiency.

The following preprocessing steps are commonly used in applied ML workflows for health classification problems:

(a) *Factor Encoding:*

Categorical variables must be converted into numerical representations before they can be processed by most machine learning algorithms. In R, variables such as *gender*, *smoking status*, and *income level* can be encoded as factors. This allows the models to correctly interpret them as non-ordinal categories rather than imposing inappropriate rank order.

(b) *Stratified Train-Test Splitting:*

To maintain the proportion of the target variable—*SUD_Status*—in both training and testing subsets, stratified sampling is essential. This is particularly important for imbalanced datasets, as it ensures balanced class representation, reduces potential bias, and enhances the generalizability of model results.

(c) *Feature Scaling:*

Continuous variables such as *BMI*, *cholesterol*, and *glucose* may vary significantly in their numeric ranges. Standardizing or normalizing these features improves the performance of algorithms that are sensitive to scale differences, such as logistic regression, support vector machines, and k-nearest neighbors. Proper scaling ensures that no single variable disproportionately influences model predictions.

ChatGPT can assist with generating the relevant R code using a structured prompt. For example:

> Using the simulated data, generate R code for advanced data preprocessing including factor encoding, stratified train-test splitting, and feature scaling for a substance use disorder prediction dataset with both categorical and continuous variables.

This prompt will return a complete R script that guides users through the key technical steps required to prepare the dataset for machine learning analysis. Within the ChatGPT interface, sample code will be generated, as shown in Fig. 8.1:

Users can then copy and paste these codes into RStudio and execute them. The same code executed in RStudio is illustrated in Fig. 8.2:

As emphasized in earlier chapters, readers should first ensure that the required packages—*caret*, *dplyr*, and *readr*—are installed using the `install.packages()` command. The diagram above illustrates the use of the RStudio script editor, where users can write, save, and modify their code. This practice of scripting is strongly encouraged throughout the book as it supports reproducibility, iterative learning, and efficient code management.

In this example, we begin by loading the necessary libraries and importing the simulated EHR dataset. Categorical variables such as *Gender*, *Income_Level*, *Smoking_Status*, and *Exercise_Level* are converted into factor variables. This step ensures that machine learning algorithms properly interpret these as categorical rather than numeric features. The target variable *SUD_Status* is also encoded as factors to denote class membership—0 for absence and 1 for presence of substance use disorder.

The dataset is then partitioned into training and testing subsets using the `createDataPartition()` function from the *caret* package. This function applies stratified sampling to maintain the class distribution of *SUD_Status* in both subsets. Such stratification is particularly important in classification tasks involving imbalanced outcomes, as it reduces sampling bias and improves the validity of model evaluation.

Subsequently, feature scaling is applied to continuous variables including *Age*, *BMI*, *Systolic_BP*, *Diastolic_BP*, *Glucose*, and *Mental_Health_Score* using the `preProcess()` function. These variables are standardized to have a mean of 0 and a standard deviation of 1. Standardization is especially important for

```r
r                                                          Copy  Edit

# Load required libraries
library(caret)
library(dplyr)
library(readr)

# Set seed for reproducibility
set.seed(123)

# Load the dataset
data <- read_csv("simulated_ehr_dataset.csv")

# Convert appropriate variables to factors
categorical_vars <- c("Gender", "Income_Level", "Smoking_Status", "Exercise_Level", "SUD_
data[categorical_vars] <- lapply(data[categorical_vars], as.factor)

# Stratified train-test split (80/20)
trainIndex <- createDataPartition(data$SUD_Status, p = 0.8, list = FALSE)
train <- data[trainIndex, ]
test <- data[-trainIndex, ]

# Identify numeric columns for scaling
numeric_vars <- c("Age", "BMI", "Systolic_BP", "Diastolic_BP", "Glucose", "Mental_Health_

# Apply standard scaling (Z-score normalization)
preProcValues <- preProcess(train[, numeric_vars], method = c("center", "scale"))

train_scaled <- train
train_scaled[, numeric_vars] <- predict(preProcValues, train[, numeric_vars])

test_scaled <- test
test_scaled[, numeric_vars] <- predict(preProcValues, test[, numeric_vars])

# Check result
str(train_scaled)
str(test_scaled)
```

Fig. 8.1 Data preprocessing steps generated by ChatGPT using the simulated dataset

algorithms sensitive to differences in feature magnitude, such as logistic regression, k-nearest neighbors, and support vector machines. As noted by Kuhn and Johnson (2013), "*Feature scaling is often a critical preprocessing step to ensure fair treatment of input variables in many machine learning algorithms.*"

Together, these preprocessing steps—factor encoding, stratified sampling, and feature scaling—produce a clean, balanced, and normalized dataset. This preparation is essential for building accurate and interpretable machine learning models to support substance use disorder prediction in real-world public health applications.

```
# Load required libraries
library(caret)
library(dplyr)
library(readr)

# Set seed for reproducibility
set.seed(123)

# Load the dataset
data <- read_csv("simulated_ehr_dataset.csv")

# Convert appropriate variables to factors
categorical_vars <- c("Gender", "Income_Level", "Smoking_Status", "Exercise_Level", "SUD_Status")
data[categorical_vars] <- lapply(data[categorical_vars], as.factor)

# Stratified train-test split (80/20)
trainIndex <- createDataPartition(data$SUD_Status, p = 0.8, list = FALSE)
train <- data[trainIndex, ]
test <- data[-trainIndex, ]

# Identify numeric columns for scaling
numeric_vars <- c("Age", "BMI", "Systolic_BP", "Diastolic_BP", "Glucose", "Mental_Health_Score", "Family_History_SUD")

# Apply standard scaling (Z-score normalization)
preProcValues <- preProcess(train[, numeric_vars], method = c("center", "scale"))

train_scaled <- train
train_scaled[, numeric_vars] <- predict(preProcValues, train[, numeric_vars])

test_scaled <- test
test_scaled[, numeric_vars] <- predict(preProcValues, test[, numeric_vars])

# Check result
str(train_scaled)
str(test_scaled)
```

Fig. 8.2 Data preprocessing steps in RStudio software interface

Logistic Regression

With the dataset properly prepared through factor encoding, stratified sampling, and feature scaling, we can now proceed to fit machine learning models to address public health research questions. As a first step, we apply a logistic regression model. This model is widely used in public health and clinical research due to its interpretability and ability to estimate the probability of a binary outcome. In this context, it serves as a useful baseline for predicting substance use disorder (*SUD_Status*) and for evaluating the relative contribution of various risk factors.

Logistic regression estimates the likelihood that an individual has substance use disorder based on a set of predictors. In this example, we include all available variables from the training dataset. These predictors cover a broad range of determinants, including:

- **Demographic characteristics:** *Age*, *Gender*, *Income_Level.*
- **Clinical indicators:** *BMI*, *Systolic_BP*, *Diastolic_BP*, *Glucose.*
- **Behavioral risk factors:** *Smoking_Status*, *Exercise_Level.*
- **Mental health indicator:** *Mental_Health_Score.*
- **Family history:** *Family_History_SUD.*

By including all predictors in the model, logistic regression enables us to assess the independent effect of each variable while controlling for the influence of others.

```
37  # Load required libraries
38  library(caret)
39  library(dplyr)
40
41  # Set seed for reproducibility
42  set.seed(123)
43
44  # Ensure SUD_Status is a factor
45  train$SUD_Status <- as.factor(train$SUD_Status)
46  test$SUD_Status <- as.factor(test$SUD_Status)
47
48  # Run logistic regression using all predictors
49  logit_model <- glm(SUD_Status ~ ., data = train, family = binomial)
50
51  # Display model coefficients
52  summary(logit_model)
53
54  # Predict on test data (probability output)
55  pred_probs <- predict(logit_model, newdata = test, type = "response")
56
57  # Convert probabilities to class labels (threshold = 0.5)
58  pred_labels <- ifelse(pred_probs > 0.5, 1, 0)
59  pred_labels <- as.factor(pred_labels)
60
61  # Confusion matrix
62  confusionMatrix(pred_labels, test$SUD_Status, positive = "1")
63
```

Fig. 8.3 Running a logistic regression model in RStudio

The R code for implementing this model was generated using the following prompt in ChatGPT:

> Write R code to run a logistic regression model using a dataset called train to predict a binary outcome SUD_Status based on all available predictors. Then, use the model to predict on a test dataset and calculate a confusion matrix. Also, show how to display the model coefficients using the summary() function. Use a set.seed command to ensure reproducible results.

The code output from ChatGPT was copied into the RStudio script editor, as illustrated in the diagram above. As emphasized in earlier chapters, using the script editor enables users to save, modify, and re-run code efficiently—facilitating a transparent and reproducible machine learning workflow.

Readers are encouraged to paste the new code into the same script file used for data preprocessing and execute it in modular blocks using the *Run* button or keyboard shortcuts. This structured and iterative approach supports experimentation, model comparison, and debugging, especially as we introduce additional machine learning models in the sections that follow.

In Fig. 8.3, the statement on **line *38*** loads the *caret* library. Although technically optional at this point—since this package was previously used during the preprocessing stage—explicitly including this line ensures that all relevant functions, such as `confusionMatrix()`, remain accessible in the R session. **Line *42*** sets the random seed using `set.seed(123)` to ensure reproducibility. This is a recommended practice whenever the analysis involves random processes such as data partitioning or probabilistic model behavior. By fixing the seed, readers can replicate the same results across different runs of the script. **Lines *45* and *46*** ensure that the target variable, *SUD_Status*, is properly encoded as a factor. This is a critical step, as classification models such as logistic regression require the outcome variable to be explicitly identified as a categorical factor with two levels representing presence and absence of substance use disorder.

R is an object-based programming language, and **line *49*** defines the logistic regression model as an object using the `glm()` function, which stands for *generalized linear model*. The model object, *logit_model*, estimates the binary outcome *SUD_Status* as a function of all other available predictors in the training dataset (*train*). The tilde symbol ~ indicates the relationship between the dependent variable and the predictors, while the period symbol `.` tells R to include all other variables except the target. The argument `family` = `binomial` specifies that the model is for a binary classification problem using the logistic link function.

In this model, predictors include:

- *Demographic variables*: *Age*, *Gender*, *Income_Level.*
- *Clinical indicators*: *BMI*, *Systolic_BP*, *Diastolic_BP*, *Glucose.*
- *Behavioral risk factors*: *Smoking_Status*, *Exercise_Level.*
- *Psychosocial indicator*: *Mental_Health_Score.*
- *Genetic risk factor*: *Family_History_SUD.*

Line *52* executes `summary(logit_model)`, which provides detailed output on the model's estimated parameters. This includes regression coefficients (in log-odds), standard errors, z-values, and associated p-values, allowing us to assess the statistical significance of each predictor in the model.

When viewed in the RStudio Console, the summary output includes:

- Estimated regression coefficients (log-odds scale).
- Standard errors for each coefficient.
- z-values and p-values for hypothesis testing,
- Model-level diagnostics such as null deviance, residual deviance, and AIC (Akaike Information Criterion).

These statistics are essential for interpreting the influence of individual predictors and assessing overall model fit. Figure 8.4 illustrates a typical example of this output as returned in RStudio, which serves as a foundation for further evaluation and comparison with other machine learning models.

Based on the regression output depicted in Fig. 8.4, several predictors in the current model reach or approach conventional levels of statistical significance. Most notably, *Family_History_SUD* demonstrates a strong and statistically significant positive association with substance use disorder ($p < 0.001$), indicating that individuals with a family history of SUD are substantially more likely to experience the condition themselves. In addition, *Income_LevelLow* ($p = 0.044$) and *Diastolic_BP* ($p = 0.008$) are statistically significant at the 0.05 level, suggesting that lower income and lower diastolic blood pressure are associated with increased odds of SUD. The predictor *Smoking_StatusNever* also approaches marginal significance

```
Call:
glm(formula = SUD_Status ~ ., family = binomial, data = train)

Coefficients:
                          Estimate Std. Error z value Pr(>|z|)
(Intercept)             -0.1461999  1.3355018  -0.109  0.91283
Age                      0.0055004  0.0080156   0.686  0.49258
GenderMale               0.0400048  0.1812265   0.221  0.82529
Income_LevelLow          0.5397084  0.2680438   2.014  0.04406 *
Income_LevelMedium       0.1294171  0.2688751   0.481  0.63028
BMI                     -0.0060304  0.0175683  -0.343  0.73141
Systolic_BP              0.0048683  0.0059029   0.825  0.40953
Diastolic_BP            -0.0235952  0.0089397  -2.639  0.00831 **
Glucose                 -0.0057178  0.0037303  -1.533  0.12532
Smoking_StatusFormer     0.1587356  0.2678625   0.593  0.55345
Smoking_StatusNever      0.4101676  0.2419715   1.695  0.09006 .
Exercise_LevelLow       -0.2591888  0.2360174  -1.098  0.27213
Exercise_LevelModerate -0.2232222  0.2389143  -0.934  0.35014
Mental_Health_Score     -0.0006845  0.0061988  -0.110  0.91207
Family_History_SUD       0.8589477  0.1914337   4.487 7.23e-06 ***
---
Signif. codes:  0 '***' 0.001 '**' 0.01 '*' 0.05 '.' 0.1 ' ' 1

(Dispersion parameter for binomial family taken to be 1)

    Null deviance: 817.47  on 800  degrees of freedom
Residual deviance: 778.20  on 786  degrees of freedom
AIC: 808.2

Number of Fisher Scoring iterations: 4
```

Fig. 8.4 Outputs from the logistic regression model (see Fig. 8.3) in RStudio

($p = 0.090$), indicating a potential trend in which individuals who have never smoked may be less likely to have SUD compared to current smokers, although this result does not meet standard significance thresholds.

Other variables—such as *Age*, *Gender*, *BMI*, *Glucose*, and *Mental_Health_Score*—have *p*-values well above 0.1, suggesting no statistically significant associations with SUD in this particular sample. Nonetheless, these predictors still contribute to the overall model structure and may be relevant in larger or alternative datasets with different population characteristics.

Despite the lack of significance for several individual predictors, logistic regression remains a valuable tool for predictive modeling. The estimated coefficients indicate how the log-odds of having substance use disorder change with a one-unit increase in each predictor, holding all other variables constant. For instance, the positive coefficient for *Family_History_SUD* reflects a notable increase in the likelihood of SUD among individuals with a familial predisposition.

In applied machine learning, model utility often depends more on predictive performance than on hypothesis testing alone. After estimating the logistic model, follow-up commands such as `predict()`, `ifelse()`, and `confusionMatrix()` are used to evaluate classification outcomes. These steps convert predicted probabilities into binary class labels using a defined threshold (typically 0.5), then compare the predicted values against the actual outcomes. RStudio returns a confusion matrix along with key performance metrics such as accuracy, sensitivity, and specificity—essential indicators of the model's ability to distinguish between individuals with and without SUD.

Lines *54–62* in the program are designed to generate and display the confusion matrix results. The corresponding output, as rendered in RStudio, is illustrated in Fig. 8.5.

Confusion Matrix

The logistic regression model achieved an *overall accuracy* of *78.9%*, indicating that it correctly classified nearly four out of five cases in the test dataset. However, this result is primarily driven by the model's strong performance on the majority class—individuals without substance use disorder (SUD). The *specificity* (true negative rate) is *98.7%*, meaning the model accurately identified nearly all individuals who did not have SUD.

In contrast, the *sensitivity* (true positive rate) is extremely low at *2.4%*, reflecting the model's inability to detect most individuals who actually had SUD. Among the few cases predicted as positive, only *33.3%* were correct, as indicated by the *positive predictive value (PPV)*. The *negative predictive value (NPV)* is *79.6%*, suggesting that when the model predicts "no SUD," it is frequently—but not always—accurate.

The *balanced accuracy*, which is the average of sensitivity and specificity, is *0.51*. This indicates that the model performs only marginally better than random guessing when both outcome classes are considered. The *kappa statistic* is *0.018*, showing very low agreement between predicted and actual classifications beyond what would be expected by chance. Additionally, the *McNemar's test p-value* is highly significant ($p < 0.00001$), suggesting that the model's classification errors are asymmetric and may be systematically biased toward the majority class.

Although the overall accuracy appears acceptable, the confusion matrix reveals a major limitation: the model fails to identify individuals with SUD, which is typically the primary concern in clinical and public health applications. This outcome underscores a common issue in predictive modeling with imbalanced datasets, where models may favor the dominant class and overlook minority outcomes.

To address this challenge and improve the model's ability to detect true positive cases, subsequent steps may include applying resampling methods (e.g., *SMOTE* or undersampling), incorporating regularization or cost-sensitive learning approaches, or testing alternative classification algorithms that are more robust to class imbalance—such as *random forest* or *gradient boosting*.

```
Confusion Matrix and Statistics

          Reference
Prediction   0   1
         0 156  40
         1   2   1

               Accuracy : 0.7889
                 95% CI : (0.7256, 0.8435)
    No Information Rate : 0.794
    P-Value [Acc > NIR] : 0.6098

                  Kappa : 0.0179

 Mcnemar's Test P-Value : 1.135e-08

            Sensitivity : 0.024390
            Specificity : 0.987342
         Pos Pred Value : 0.333333
         Neg Pred Value : 0.795918
             Prevalence : 0.206030
         Detection Rate : 0.005025
   Detection Prevalence : 0.015075
      Balanced Accuracy : 0.505866

       'Positive' Class : 1
```

Fig. 8.5 Confusion matrix from the logistic regression model (see Fig. 8.3) in RStudio

Decision Tree

In addition to logistic regression, decision trees provide an alternative modeling approach for identifying key predictors of substance use disorder (SUD) and evaluating classification performance. Unlike logistic regression, decision trees do not require assumptions about linear relationships among variables. Instead, they generate interpretable "if–then" rules through a process known as recursive partitioning (El-Sofany et al., 2024). These rules split the data based on threshold values of

```r
# Load necessary libraries
library(rpart)
library(rpart.plot)
library(caret)

# Set seed for reproducibility
set.seed(123)

# Ensure the target variable is a factor
train$SUD_Status <- as.factor(train$SUD_Status)
test$SUD_Status <- as.factor(test$SUD_Status)

# Train a decision tree model using all predictors
tree_model <- rpart(SUD_Status ~ ., data = train, method = "class")

# Visualize the tree
rpart.plot(tree_model, type = 3, extra = 104, fallen.leaves = TRUE)

# Generate predictions on test data
tree_predictions <- predict(tree_model, newdata = test, type = "class")

# Evaluate model performance using confusion matrix
confusionMatrix(tree_predictions, test$SUD_Status, positive = "1")
```

Fig. 8.6 Running a decision tree (DT) model in RStudio

predictor variables, allowing users to easily visualize the decision-making process. Decision trees have been widely used in public health research to identify behavioral and clinical risk factors (Mohan et al., 2019).

To implement this approach, we used the following prompt in ChatGPT:

> Write R code to apply a decision tree model in R using a dataset called 'train' to predict a binary outcome variable called SUD_Status. Use all available predictors, generate predictions on a test set, evaluate performance using a confusion matrix, and visualize the tree. Use a set.seed command to ensure reproducible results.

ChatGPT generated the corresponding R code, which was copied and executed in RStudio as part of our machine learning workflow (see Fig. 8.6). This implementation demonstrates how decision trees can be applied to SUD prediction in a transparent and reproducible manner.

Beside the *caret* package, two additional libraries—*rpart* and *rpart.plot*—are required to implement and visualize a decision tree model in R. The model object, *tree_model*, is created using the `rpart()` function, which stands for *recursive partitioning*. This function builds a classification tree to predict whether a patient has substance use disorder (*SUD_Status*) based on all available predictors in the training dataset (`data = train`). The tilde symbol ~ denotes "a function of," and the period . following the tilde includes all other variables in the dataset as predictors. The argument `method = "class"` specifies that the model is used for classification rather than regression.

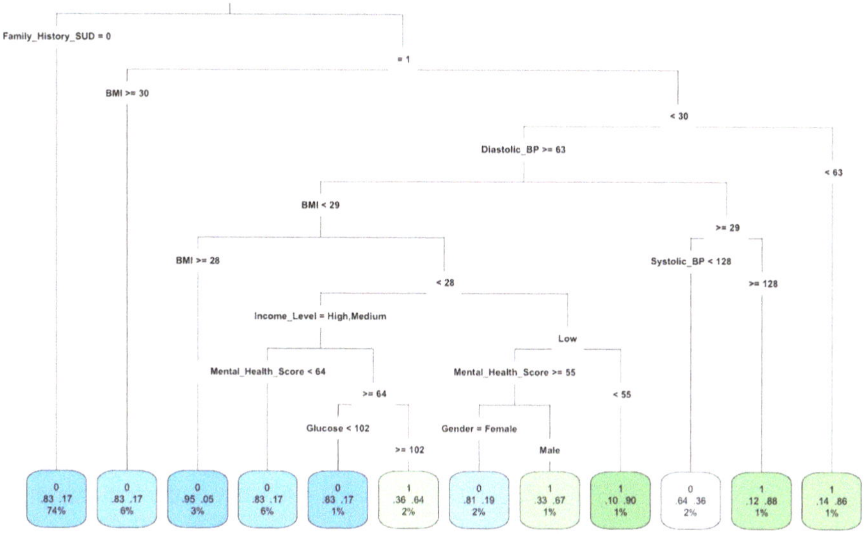

Fig. 8.7 A decision tree (DT) diagram produced in RStudio

Unlike logistic regression, decision trees do not produce individual coefficients for each predictor. Instead, the model identifies threshold values that best split the data to distinguish between outcome classes. This generates a set of intuitive "if–then" decision rules. A key strength of decision trees lies in their interpretability—their hierarchical structure makes it easy to trace the logic behind each classification outcome.

The `rpart.plot()` function is used to visualize the resulting tree structure, providing a clear and accessible summary of how decisions are made. In RStudio, the visual output from `rpart.plot()` appears as shown in Fig. 8.7, illustrating how the model segments patients into different risk categories for SUD based on combinations of predictor variables.

Interpretation of the Tree Diagram

The decision tree diagram for predicting substance use disorder (SUD) identifies *family history of SUD* as the most influential predictor, with the first split dividing individuals based on the presence or absence of such a history. Among those *without* a family history, individuals with a *body mass index (BMI)* $\geq$ *30* are consistently classified as not having SUD. Additional splits based on *BMI*, *income level*, *mental health score*, and *glucose level* further refine the risk classifications within this group.

For individuals *with* a family history of SUD, the model relies on variables such as *diastolic blood pressure*, *BMI*, *systolic blood pressure*, and *mental health score* to distinguish between higher- and lower-risk subgroups. Several terminal nodes predict SUD for a small proportion of individuals, with the highest predicted probability of SUD (up to *23%*) observed among those with a family history, *low diastolic blood pressure*, and *male gender*.

Overall, the tree highlights how *family history*, *behavioral health indicators*, and *cardiovascular measurements* jointly contribute to identifying individuals at elevated risk for substance use disorder. This structure provides a transparent and interpretable framework for understanding how different combinations of health and demographic factors influence classification outcomes.

Confusion Matrix

The `confusionMatrix()` function is used to compare the predicted class labels generated by the decision tree model with the actual outcomes in the test dataset. It returns key performance metrics, including *accuracy*, *sensitivity*, *specificity*, and *predictive values*, providing a comprehensive view of the model's classification performance.

These metrics can be directly compared to those obtained from the logistic regression model to assess which approach more effectively identifies individuals with substance use disorder. In particular, sensitivity and positive predictive value are especially important when evaluating model performance in imbalanced datasets where identifying true cases is a central concern.

In RStudio, the output shown in Fig. 8.8 is generated after executing **line *83*** (`tree_predictions <- predict(...)`) and **line *86*** (`confusionMatrix(...)`). This evaluation step is critical not only for assessing overall accuracy but also for determining the model's effectiveness in detecting true SUD cases—a primary objective in clinical and public health applications.

Confusion Matrix Interpretation

The decision tree model achieved an *accuracy* of *74.9%*, indicating that it correctly classified approximately three-quarters of the test cases. However, this overall performance is primarily driven by the model's strong ability to identify individuals *without* substance use disorder (SUD), as reflected by a high *specificity* of *92.4%*. In contrast, the *sensitivity* is markedly low at *7.3%*, suggesting that the model failed to detect the vast majority of true SUD cases.

The *positive predictive value (PPV)* is *20%*, meaning that only one in five individuals predicted to have SUD actually had the condition. The *negative predictive value (NPV)* is higher at *79.3%*, indicating that the model is more reliable in ruling out SUD than in confirming it.

```
Confusion Matrix and Statistics

          Reference
Prediction   0   1
         0 146  38
         1  12   3

               Accuracy : 0.7487
                 95% CI : (0.6825, 0.8074)
    No Information Rate : 0.794
    P-Value [Acc > NIR] : 0.949322

                  Kappa : -0.0036

 Mcnemar's Test P-Value : 0.000407

            Sensitivity : 0.07317
            Specificity : 0.92405
         Pos Pred Value : 0.20000
         Neg Pred Value : 0.79348
             Prevalence : 0.20603
         Detection Rate : 0.01508
   Detection Prevalence : 0.07538
      Balanced Accuracy : 0.49861

       'Positive' Class : 1
```

Fig. 8.8 Confusion matrix from the decision tree (DT) model (see Fig. 8.6) in RStudio

The *balanced accuracy*, which averages sensitivity and specificity, is *49.9%*, implying that the model performs no better than random guessing when both classes are considered equally. The *kappa statistic* is *−0.0036*, indicating no meaningful agreement between predicted and actual classifications beyond chance. Additionally, the *McNemar's test p-value* is statistically significant ($p = 0.0004$), suggesting that the model's prediction errors are not randomly distributed and may reflect bias toward the majority class.

While decision trees provide clear interpretability through their visual structure and if–then rules, this example highlights a key limitation: poor detection of

```
# Train the decision tree with max depth = 4
tree_model2 <- rpart(SUD_Status ~ .,
                     data = train,
                     method = "class",
                     control = rpart.control(maxdepth = 4))

# Visualize the tree
rpart.plot(tree_model2,
           type = 3,
           extra = 104,
           cex = 1,
           tweak = 0.7,
           compress = TRUE,
           box.palette = "BuGn",
           fallen.leaves = TRUE)
```

Fig. 8.9 R scripts to visualize a 4-layer decision tree in RStudio

minority-class outcomes in imbalanced datasets. Compared to logistic regression, the decision tree model underperformed in identifying high-risk individuals. To improve performance, future iterations may benefit from applying rebalancing techniques (e.g., *SMOTE*, undersampling), incorporating ensemble methods (e.g., *random forest*, *gradient boosting*), or tuning model parameters.

**Special note:* For educational and visualization purposes, it is often helpful to adjust the structure and appearance of the decision tree diagram to enhance clarity. One common adjustment is to limit the *depth* of the tree—for example, to four or five levels—using the `maxdepth` parameter within the `rpart.control()` function. This helps prevent overfitting and simplifies interpretation, particularly during instruction. Additionally, the *font size* of the plot can be increased using the `cex` and `tweak` arguments in the `rpart.plot()` function, making the diagram more readable when presenting to audiences or embedding in course materials. The R code provided in Fig. 8.9 demonstrates how to apply these controls to generate a concise and visually accessible decision tree suitable for teaching purposes:

Figure 8.10 shows the resulting diagram:

Random Forest

As introduced in Chap. 4, *random forest* is an ensemble learning method that builds on the decision tree approach. Random forest models are widely applied in healthcare analytics, including the classification of patient outcomes such as the risk of substance use disorder (SUD). Instead of relying on a single decision tree, the random forest algorithm constructs an ensemble of trees, each trained on a bootstrapped sample of the training dataset (Shah et al., 2020). Final predictions

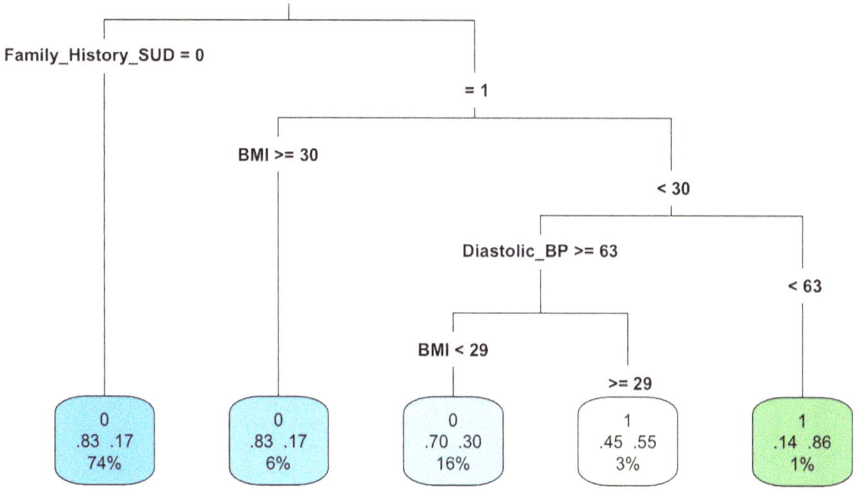

Fig. 8.10 R scripts to visualize a 4-layer decision tree in RStudio

are generated through *majority voting* across trees, which enhances model robustness and reduces the risk of overfitting (Breiman, 2001).

In this example, we applied a random forest model to classify *SUD_Status* using all available predictors in the dataset. These include demographic characteristics, behavioral risk factors, clinical indicators, and mental health measures. To initiate the modeling process, we used the following prompt in ChatGPT:

> Write R code to apply a random forest model in R using a dataset called 'train' to predict a binary outcome variable called SUD_Status. Use all available predictors, generate predictions on a test set, and evaluate performance using a confusion matrix. When using predict, no need to specify type. Then ensure the predictions are converted to binary levels (1 or 0) rather than probabilities by using the ifelse statement.

ChatGPT generated the corresponding R code, which was then copied into the RStudio script editor. The code was executed to fit the model, generate predictions on the test set, and evaluate classification performance using a confusion matrix (see Fig. 8.11):

Interpretation

The R script demonstrates how to apply a random forest model to classify whether a patient has substance use disorder (*SUD_Status*) using all available predictors in the training dataset. After loading the necessary libraries (*randomForest* and *caret*), the script sets a random seed to ensure reproducibility and converts the outcome variable *SUD_Status* into a factor to ensure compatibility with classification functions.

```
# Load required libraries
library(randomForest)
library(caret)

# Set seed for reproducibility
set.seed(123)

# Ensure the outcome variable is a factor
train$SUD_Status <- as.factor(train$SUD_Status)
test$SUD_Status <- as.factor(test$SUD_Status)

# Train the random forest model using all predictors
rf_model <- randomForest(SUD_Status ~ ., data = train, ntree = 500, importance = TRUE)

# Generate predictions on the test set
rf_pred <- predict(rf_model, newdata = test)

# Convert predictions to binary levels (0 or 1) if needed
# (This step is included for consistency; rf_pred is already a factor with levels 0 and 1)
rf_pred_binary <- ifelse(rf_pred == "1", 1, 0)
rf_pred_binary <- as.factor(rf_pred_binary)

# Evaluate performance using a confusion matrix
confusionMatrix(rf_pred_binary, test$SUD_Status, positive = "1")

```

Fig. 8.11 Running a random forest (RF) model in RStudio

The `randomForest()` function is then used to train the model, specifying *ntree* = *500* to grow 500 decision trees. The argument *importance* = *TRUE* is included to enable calculation of variable importance scores, which can later be used to assess the relative contribution of each predictor. Predictions on the test dataset are generated using the `predict()` function. Although the output is already in factor format, an `ifelse()` statement is applied to explicitly convert the predictions to binary values (0 or 1), ensuring consistency with earlier models and enabling comparison across methods.

Model performance is evaluated using the `confusionMatrix()` function, which compares the predicted class labels with the actual outcomes in the test set. It returns key metrics such as *accuracy*, *sensitivity*, *specificity*, and *balanced accuracy*, providing a comprehensive view of the model's classification capabilities.

The confusion matrix output, as displayed in RStudio, is shown in Fig. 8.12.

The random forest model achieved an *accuracy* of *80.4%*. As with the decision tree model discussed above, this performance is largely driven by the model's ability to correctly identify individuals *without* substance use disorder (SUD), as reflected in a high *specificity* of *99.4%*. In contrast, the *sensitivity* is only *7.3%*, indicating that the model failed to detect the vast majority of true SUD cases.

On the other hand, the *positive predictive value (PPV)* is *75%*, suggesting that three out of four individuals predicted to have SUD actually did have the condition. The *negative predictive value (NPV)* is *80.5%*, meaning the model was more reliable in ruling out SUD than confirming it.

The *balanced accuracy*, which averages sensitivity and specificity, is *53.3%*, suggesting the model performs only slightly better than random guessing when both classes are weighted equally. The *kappa statistic* is *0.1004*, indicating weak

```
Confusion Matrix and Statistics

          Reference
Prediction   0   1
         0 157  38
         1   1   3

               Accuracy : 0.804
                 95% CI : (0.742, 0.8568)
    No Information Rate : 0.794
    P-Value [Acc > NIR] : 0.4026

                  Kappa : 0.1004

 Mcnemar's Test P-Value : 8.185e-09

            Sensitivity : 0.07317
            Specificity : 0.99367
         Pos Pred Value : 0.75000
         Neg Pred Value : 0.80513
             Prevalence : 0.20603
         Detection Rate : 0.01508
   Detection Prevalence : 0.02010
      Balanced Accuracy : 0.53342

       'Positive' Class : 1
```

Fig. 8.12 Confusion matrix from the random forest (RF) model (in Fig. 8.11) in RStudio

agreement between predicted and actual classifications beyond chance. The *McNemar's test p-value* is statistically significant ($p < 0.00001$), further confirming that prediction errors are not randomly distributed and that the model is likely biased toward the majority class.

Although the model achieves high overall accuracy, this is driven almost entirely by correct identification of non-SUD cases. Like the logistic regression and decision tree models, the random forest model continues to struggle with detecting true cases of SUD due to the imbalanced nature of the dataset. However, the relatively high

PPV indicates that when the model does predict SUD, it is often correct. These results highlight the persistent challenge of working with imbalanced health data, where the minority class—in this case, individuals with SUD—is underrepresented and difficult to detect.

Importance Rankings

One of the key advantages of the random forest algorithm is its ability to generate *variable importance rankings*, which identify the predictors that contribute most significantly to the model's performance. This capability is particularly valuable in public health contexts, where understanding the relative influence of behavioral, demographic, and clinical factors can inform targeted prevention and intervention strategies. While random forests are generally less interpretable than single decision trees, their superior predictive performance and resistance to overfitting often make them a preferred choice when accuracy is prioritized.

In RStudio, the `importance()` function provides a summary of each variable's importance based on two key metrics: *MeanDecreaseAccuracy* and *MeanDecreaseGini*. These measures reflect the extent to which each predictor improves classification accuracy and contributes to node purity within the ensemble of trees. The `varImpPlot()` function generates a visual representation of the top predictors ranked by importance, offering an accessible way to identify which features most strongly influence the model's predictions.

Additionally, the `plot()` function can be used to visualize the *out-of-bag (OOB) error rate* across the growing number of trees in the model. A flattening error curve suggests that the model is converging and that additional trees are contributing little to further accuracy gains—an indication of model stability.

The R code and output related to variable importance for the random forest model (*rf_model*) are shown in Fig. 8.13.

According to the results, the top predictors by *MeanDecreaseAccuracy* are *Family_History_SUD* (5.97), *Income_Level* (3.18), *Exercise_Level* (0.70), *Glucose* (0.48), and *BMI* (0.30). In terms of *MeanDecreaseGini*, the highest-ranked predictors are *Glucose* (40.30), *Mental_Health_Score* (39.99), *BMI* (39.14), *Systolic_BP* (33.49), and *Age* (32.91). Taken together, these rankings highlight several overlapping variables—most notably, *Family_History_SUD*, *Glucose*, *Mental_Health_Score*, *BMI*, and blood pressure measures—as key contributors to the model's predictive performance. These results suggest that both clinical indicators (such as glucose levels and blood pressure) and behavioral or psychosocial factors (including mental health and family history) are important for identifying individuals at risk for substance use disorder. The varImpPlot(rf_model) produces the plot for visualization that is shown in Fig. 8.14:

Using the *plot(rf_model)* function, users can display the out-of-bag (OOB) error rate across the number of trees, providing insight into whether the model's performance has stabilized. The output is generated in RStudio as depicted in Fig. 8.15:

```
importance(rf_model)

varImpPlot(rf_model)

plot(rf_model)
```

```
> importance(rf_model)
                             0            1 MeanDecreaseAccuracy MeanDecreaseGini
Age                 -1.2401435 -1.039777755           -1.5893735        32.909984
Gender              -0.1445368 -1.254281271           -0.8252930         5.375670
Income_Level         1.1442167  4.498524850            3.1815708        10.031138
BMI                  0.1039991  0.444529178            0.2957311        39.139411
Systolic_BP         -3.1235267 -1.033456499           -3.1474952        33.485844
Diastolic_BP        -1.5842615  0.583854516           -1.1028612        32.557119
Glucose              0.5302954  0.003225538            0.4838113        40.303095
Smoking_Status      -1.4601857 -2.126294425           -2.2487128         9.447392
Exercise_Level       1.5711515 -1.350164126            0.6950157        10.507751
Mental_Health_Score -2.6325760 -3.679128190           -4.1357227        39.998754
Family_History_SUD   2.6779439  7.593343533            5.9714202         8.259619
```

Fig. 8.13 Displaying the importance of feature variables in the random forest (RF) model (in Fig. 8.11) in RStudio

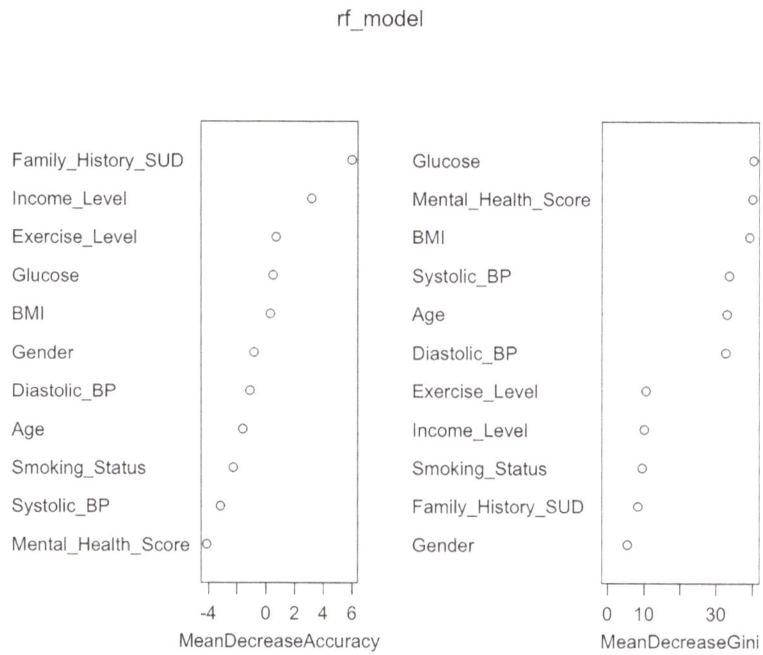

Fig. 8.14 A graphical display to compare the importance of feature variables in the random forest (RF) model (in Fig. 8.11) in RStudio

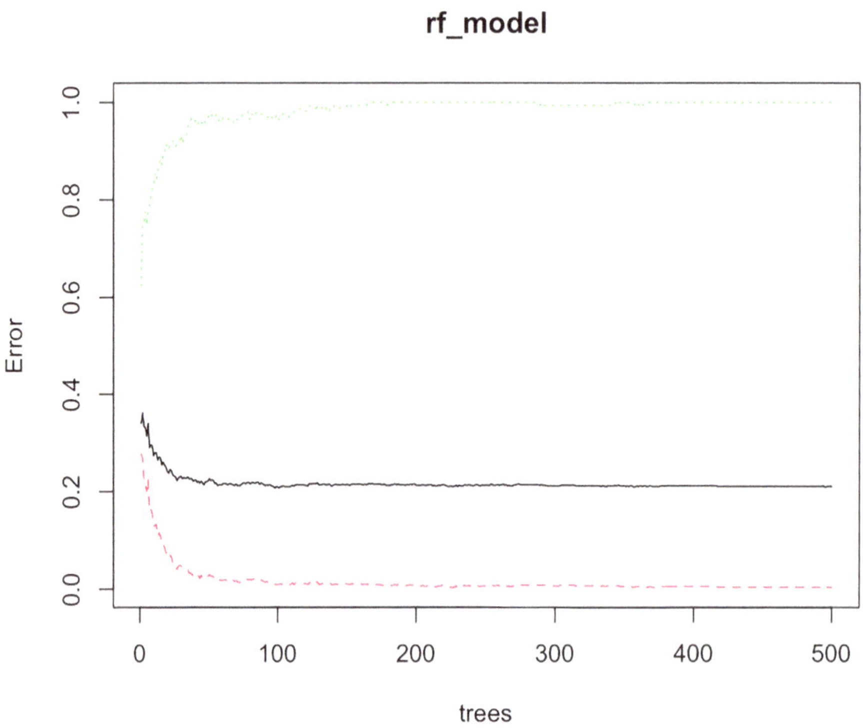

Fig. 8.15 A graph to show the out-of-bag (OOB) error rate as the number of trees increases in the random forest (RF) model (in Fig. 8.11) in RStudio

The `plot(rf_model)` function in R displays the out-of-bag (OOB) error rate as the number of trees increases in a random forest model. The resulting plot typically includes three curves, each representing a different class-specific or overall error rate:

(a) ***Black Curve—Overall OOB Error Rate***
This curve shows the average classification error across all classes as more trees are added. It provides a general indication of the model's overall performance. A declining or flattening black curve suggests that model accuracy has stabilized and that adding more trees does not result in significant improvement.

(b) ***Red Curve—Class 0 (No SUD) OOB Error***
This curve tracks the classification error for the negative class (patients without SUD). It reflects how often non-SUD cases are misclassified. A consistently low red curve indicates strong model performance in identifying non-SUD cases, which is typical in imbalanced datasets.

(c) ***Green Curve—Class 1 (SUD) OOB Error***
This curve represents the error rate for the positive class (patients with SUD). It indicates how frequently individuals with SUD are misclassified. In many health-related datasets, where the positive class is underrepresented, the green

curve tends to remain higher—highlighting the model's difficulty in correctly identifying minority cases.

Model Evaluation and Visualization

At this stage, the analyst has several options for evaluating and refining the machine learning (ML) models. A key step involves comparing evaluation metrics—such as *accuracy*, *sensitivity*, *specificity*, and *AUC*—produced by the confusion matrices of the three models. This comparison helps determine which model is best suited for the agency's goal of predicting the risk of substance use disorder (SUD) based on patients' demographic and behavioral characteristics. The results can also inform targeted recommendations for individuals at higher risk, thereby supporting prevention and treatment strategies.

To facilitate this evaluation, we used ChatGPT to generate code for a systematic comparison of the three models. To ensure fairness and consistency, all models were re-run using the same training and testing datasets within a unified workflow. An effective prompt for this task was:

> Write R code to fit and evaluate logistic regression, decision tree, and random forest models using the same training and test data. Collect performance metrics (e.g., accuracy, sensitivity, specificity, AUC) for each model and display them side by side for comparison.

The R code generated by ChatGPT was copied into RStudio and executed to complete the evaluation sequence, as shown in Fig. 8.16.

The R script (see Fig. 8.16) performs a complete end-to-end workflow for training and evaluating three machine learning models—logistic regression, decision tree, and random forest—to predict substance use disorder (SUD) using a simulated EHR dataset. It begins by loading the necessary libraries (*caret*, *rpart*, *randomForest*, *pROC*) and setting a random seed to ensure reproducibility. The dataset is read from a CSV file, and the target variable (*SUD_Status*) is converted into a factor suitable for classification. Using stratified sampling, the data is split into training (80%) and testing (20%) sets while preserving class proportions. The script then fits three models: a logistic regression using all predictors, a decision tree constrained to a maximum depth of four, and a random forest with 500 trees and variable importance tracking. For each model, it generates predicted probabilities and class labels on the test set. A custom evaluation function computes key metrics—accuracy, sensitivity, specificity, balanced accuracy, and AUC—for each model. These metrics are then combined into a summary table, allowing for direct comparison of model performance. The final output is a printed table displaying the evaluation results, supporting interpretation of which model best identifies individuals at risk for SUD (see Fig. 8.17):

As shown in Fig. 8.17 in the RStudio results, if we focus on metrics derived from the confusion matrix, the random forest model outperformed both the decision tree and logistic regression models in terms of overall *accuracy*, *sensitivity*, *specificity*,

```r
############################################################
## 1.  Setup
############################################################
library(caret)        # data splitting & performance
library(rpart)        # decision tree
library(rpart.plot)   # (optional) tree plot
library(randomForest) # random forest
library(pROC)         # AUC / ROC curves

set.seed(123)         # reproducibility

############################################################
## 2.  Read data  &  stratified split  (80/20)
############################################################
data <- read.csv("simulated_ehr_dataset.csv")

# ensure target is factor
data$SUD_Status <- as.factor(data$SUD_Status)

idx  <- createDataPartition(data$SUD_Status, p = 0.8, list = FALSE)
train <- data[idx, ]
test  <- data[-idx, ]

############################################################
## 3.  Fit three models
############################################################
#--- (a) Logistic regression --------------------------------
logit_mod <- glm(SUD_Status ~ ., data = train, family = binomial)

#--- (b) Decision tree (depth capped at 4) ------------------
tree_mod  <- rpart(
  SUD_Status ~ ., data = train, method = "class",
  control = rpart.control(maxdepth = 4)
)

#--- (c) Random forest --------------------------------------
rf_mod     <- randomForest(SUD_Status ~ ., data = train,
                          ntree = 500, importance = TRUE)

```

Fig. 8.16 Comparing three ML models: logistic regression, decision tree (DT) and random forest (RF) in RStudio

and *balanced accuracy* for detecting substance use disorder (SUD). These contingency matrix metrics provide a side-by-side evaluation of classification performance across the three models. However, the *area under the ROC curve (AUC)* was highest for the logistic regression model, suggesting that it may offer better overall discrimination between positive and negative cases across a range of probability thresholds.

```r
#############################################################
## 3.  Fit three models
#############################################################
#--- (a) Logistic regression --------------------------------
logit_mod <- glm(SUD_Status ~ ., data = train, family = binomial)

#--- (b) Decision tree (depth capped at 4) ------------------
tree_mod  <- rpart(
  SUD_Status ~ ., data = train, method = "class",
  control = rpart.control(maxdepth = 4)
)

#--- (c) Random forest --------------------------------------
rf_mod    <- randomForest(SUD_Status ~ ., data = train,
                          ntree = 500, importance = TRUE)

#############################################################
## 4.  Generate predictions & probabilities
#############################################################
# Positive class is "1"
# Logistic
logit_prob <- predict(logit_mod, newdata = test, type = "response")
logit_pred <- factor(ifelse(logit_prob > 0.5, 1, 0), levels = c(0,1))

# Decision tree
tree_prob  <- predict(tree_mod, newdata = test, type = "prob")[, "1"]
tree_pred  <- predict(tree_mod, newdata = test, type = "class")

# Random forest
rf_prob    <- predict(rf_mod,  newdata = test, type = "prob")[, "1"]
rf_pred    <- predict(rf_mod,  newdata = test)  # already factor 0/1

#############################################################
## 5.  Evaluate each model
#############################################################
eval_metrics <- function(truth, pred, prob) {
  cm <- confusionMatrix(pred, truth, positive = "1")
  data.frame(
    Accuracy  = cm$overall["Accuracy"],
    Sens      = cm$byClass["Sensitivity"],
    Spec      = cm$byClass["Specificity"],
    BalAcc    = cm$byClass["Balanced Accuracy"],
    AUC       = auc(truth, prob)[1]
  )
}

results <- rbind(
  Logistic      = eval_metrics(test$SUD_Status, logit_pred, logit_prob),
  DecisionTree  = eval_metrics(test$SUD_Status, tree_pred,  tree_prob),
  RandomForest  = eval_metrics(test$SUD_Status, rf_pred,    rf_prob)
)
```

Fig. 8.16 (continued)

```
> ################################################################
> ## 6.  Display comparison table
> ################################################################
> print(round(results, 4))
             Accuracy   Sens   Spec BalAcc    AUC
Logistic       0.7889 0.0244 0.9873 0.5059 0.6110
DecisionTree   0.7739 0.0244 0.9684 0.4964 0.6089
RandomForest   0.7990 0.0488 0.9937 0.5212 0.6004
```

Fig. 8.17 A comparison table of three ML models: logistic regression, decision tree (DT), and random forest (RF) in RStudio

```
################################################################
## 7.  (Optional) plot ROC curves on same graph
################################################################
plot(roc(test$SUD_Status, logit_prob), col = "black", lwd = 2, main = "ROC Comparison")
plot(roc(test$SUD_Status, tree_prob),  col = "blue",  lwd = 2, add = TRUE)
plot(roc(test$SUD_Status, rf_prob),    col = "green", lwd = 2, add = TRUE)
legend("bottomright",
       legend = c("Logistic", "Decision Tree", "Random Forest"),
       col    = c("black", "blue", "green"), lwd = 2)

################################################################
# End of script
################################################################

```

Fig. 8.18 Plotting ROC curves for three ML models: logistic regression, decision tree (DT), and random forest (RF) in RStudio

Importantly, all three models demonstrated low sensitivity, underscoring the challenge of identifying true SUD cases—likely due to class imbalance in the dataset. To address this limitation, future work could incorporate resampling techniques (e.g., *SMOTE*) or more advanced ensemble algorithms (e.g., *XGBoost*) to improve detection of minority-class cases while preserving interpretability. These approaches, however, are beyond the scope of this book.

Given the evaluation results, one analyst might favor the random forest model for its consistently strong performance across multiple metrics, while another might prefer the logistic regression model due to its higher AUC and interpretability. To further visualize the comparative performance of these models, the R code in Fig. 8.18 plots ROC curves for all three models on a single graph. This visualization provides a clear graphical summary of each model's ability to distinguish between SUD and non-SUD cases across varying classification thresholds.

The results are shown in Fig. 8.19:

The difference in the shape of the ROC (Receiver Operating Characteristic) curves—particularly the stepped versus smooth appearance—reflects how each model generates predicted probabilities for the positive class, which the ROC curve uses to compute sensitivity (true positive rate) and specificity (false positive rate) across a range of thresholds.

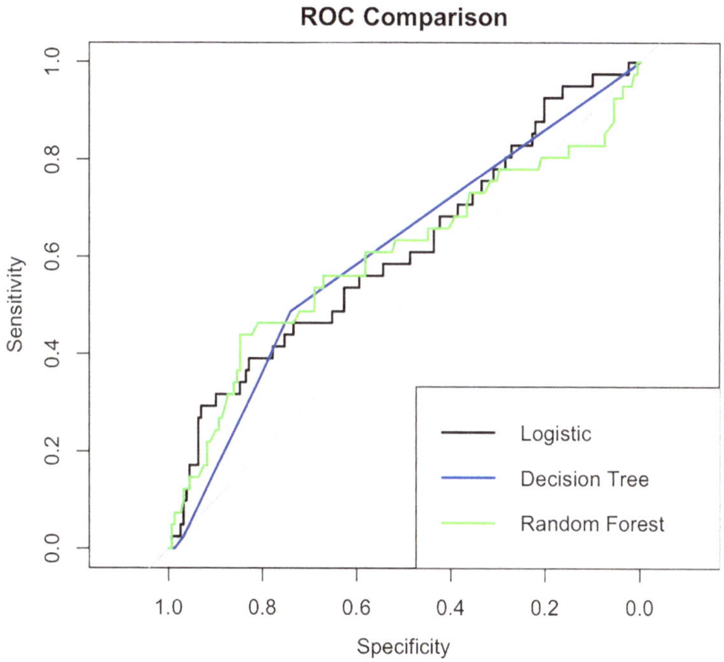

Fig. 8.19 A graph to compare the ROC curves for three models: logistic regression, decision tree (DT), and random forest (RF)

Summary

This chapter built upon the supervised learning foundation introduced in Chap. 4 by guiding readers through additional analytic steps essential for applied practice in public health and clinical settings. Readers learned how to implement and compare multiple machine learning algorithms—including logistic regression, decision trees, and random forests—using a simulated EHR dataset focused on predicting substance use disorder (SUD). The chapter also covered key evaluation techniques, such as confusion matrix metrics and ROC analysis, to assess model performance and interpret results meaningfully. Finally, the integration of generative AI tools, such as ChatGPT, illustrated how emerging technologies can support and streamline analytical workflows while maintaining scientific rigor and reproducibility.

Discussion Questions

1. Why might a public health practitioner choose a decision tree over logistic regression?
2. How would you interpret the variable importance rankings in a random forest model?
3. What are the potential pitfalls in using accuracy as the only metric for model performance?
4. How can overfitting be detected and reduced in classification models?

References

Adler-Milstein, J., Holmgren, A. J., Kralovec, P., Worzala, C., Searcy, T., & Patel, V. (2017). Electronic health record adoption in US hospitals: the emergence of a digital "advanced use" divide. *Journal of the American Medical Informatics Association, 24*(6), 1142–1148. https://academic.oup.com/jamia/article-abstract/24/6/1142/4091350

Breiman, L. (2001). Random forests. *Machine Learning, 45*(1), 5–32. https://doi.org/10.1023/A:1010933404324

Chen, J. H., & Asch, S. M. (2017). Machine learning and prediction in medicine—Beyond the peak of inflated expectations. *New England Journal of Medicine, 376*(26), 2507–2509. https://www.nejm.org/doi/10.1056/NEJMp1702071

El-Sofany, H., Bouallegue, B., & El-Latif, Y. M. A. (2024). A proposed technique for predicting heart disease using machine learning algorithms and an explainable AI method. *Scientific Reports, 14*, 23277. https://doi.org/10.1038/s41598-024-74656-2

Goldstein, B. A., Navar, A. M., Pencina, M. J., & Ioannidis, J. P. (2017). Opportunities and challenges in developing risk prediction models with electronic health records data: A systematic review. *Journal of the American Medical Informatics Association, 24*(1), 198–208. https://academic.oup.com/jamia/article/24/1/198/2631444

Kuhn, M., & Johnson, K. (2013). *Applied predictive modeling* (Vol. 26, p. 13). New York: Springer. https://link.springer.com/book/10.1007/978-1-4614-6849-3

Leung, R. C. (2012). Health information technology and dynamic capabilities. *Health Care Management Review, 37*(1), 43–53. https://journals.lww.com/hcmrjournal/abstract/2012/01000/health_information_technology_and_dynamic.6.aspx

Menachemi, N., & Collum, T. H. (2011). Benefits and drawbacks of electronic health record systems. Risk management and healthcare policy, 47–55. https://www.tandfonline.com/doi/full/10.2147/RMHP.S12985

Mohan, S., Thirumalai, C., & Srivastava, G. (2019). Effective heart disease prediction using hybrid machine learning techniques. *IEEE Access, 7*, 81542–81554. https://doi.org/10.1109/ACCESS.2019.2923707

Mokdad, A. H., Ballestros, K., Echko, M., Glenn, S., Olsen, H. E., Mullany, E., et al. (2018). The state of US health, 1990–2016: Burden of diseases, injuries, and risk factors among US states. *JAMA, 319*(14), 1444–1472. https://jamanetwork.com/journals/jama/fullarticle/2678018

Rajkomar, A., Dean, J., & Kohane, I. (2019). Machine learning in medicine. *New England Journal of Medicine, 380*(14), 1347–1358. https://www.nejm.org/doi/full/10.1056/NEJMra1814259

Shah, S. A., Brown, P., Gimeno, H., Lin, J. P., & McClelland, V. M. (2020). Application of machine learning using decision trees for prognosis of deep brain stimulation of globus pallidus internus for children with dystonia. *Frontiers in neurology, 11*, 825. https://www.frontiersin.org/journals/neurology/articles/10.3389/fneur.2020.00825/full

Chapter 9
Explainability and Reproducibility in Machine Learning

Learning Objectives
By the end of this chapter, students will be able to:

1. **Define** explainability and its importance in health-related machine learning (ML) applications.
2. **Apply** Local Interpretable Model-Agnostic Explanations (LIME) to interpret model predictions.
3. **Evaluate** the challenges of model reproducibility when using generative AI tools such as ChatGPT.
4. **Develop** critical thinking skills to balance predictive performance and interpretability in public health decision-making.

Why Explainability Matters

As discussed in Chap. 8, machine learning (ML) models such as logistic regression, decision trees, and random forests offer valuable tools for predicting health outcomes. However, their successful integration into clinical and public health settings often depends on one critical element: explainability. Explainability refers to the degree to which humans can understand the reasoning behind a model's prediction or decision (Doshi-Velez & Kim, 2017). In healthcare—where decisions directly affect diagnosis, treatment, and policy—transparent models are not merely beneficial; they are increasingly essential. Regulatory bodies now frequently mandate interpretability for AI systems used in clinical applications (Holzinger et al., 2017).

Explainability's importance extends well beyond compliance. It plays a central role in trust and adoption. Empirical studies examining the influence of explainable

Supplementary Information The online version contains supplementary material available at https://doi.org/10.1007/978-3-032-08677-8_9.

R. Leung, *Leveraging GenAI for Machine Learning Education in Public Health*,
https://doi.org/10.1007/978-3-032-08677-8_9

AI on physician trust report mixed findings: while approximately 50% of studies show increased trust, about 20% observe both positive and negative effects. These mixed results suggest that explainability alone is not enough—the quality, clarity, and clinical relevance of explanations are equally important. Healthcare professionals often evaluate AI recommendations by comparing them to established "gold standards" such as randomized controlled trials. When explainability complements clinicians' judgment and experience, it enables more informed and confident decision-making.

The high-stakes nature of medical decision-making further heightens the demand for meaningful explainability. Failures of AI in healthcare can have serious clinical consequences and risk undermining public confidence. Thus, explainability must be embedded alongside transparency, usability, and user education. Together, these factors contribute to building healthcare professionals' trust in AI systems and ensuring alignment with clinical workflows and patient safety goals.

Some models are inherently interpretable. Decision trees offer intuitive "if–then" logic, and logistic regression provides understandable coefficients and odds ratios. In contrast, more complex models like random forests, gradient boosting, and neural networks are often considered black boxes (Lipton, 2018). To bridge this gap, post-hoc explanation tools such as LIME (Ribeiro et al., 2016) and SHAP (Lundberg & Lee, 2017) have gained prominence. These model-agnostic techniques are increasingly used in healthcare to make high-performing models interpretable, allowing practitioners to leverage predictive accuracy without sacrificing transparency.

Conceptual Framework of Explainability

Explainability in machine learning (ML) is a multidimensional concept that goes beyond simply categorizing models as interpretable or not. Especially in healthcare, where decisions may carry life-altering consequences, explainability must be understood through a more nuanced framework. Several important distinctions—such as global versus local, intrinsic versus post-hoc, model-agnostic versus model-specific, and stakeholder-centered approaches—inform how we design and implement explainable ML systems in practice.

The first key distinction is between *global* and *local* interpretability. Global interpretability refers to understanding a model's behavior across the entire dataset. It answers questions such as which features are most influential overall—e.g., feature importance rankings from a random forest model can identify predictors like age, blood pressure, or family history as dominant in cardiovascular risk estimation (Breiman, 2001). By contrast, local interpretability focuses on why the model made a specific prediction for an individual case. Techniques like LIME offer case-specific insights by approximating the model with a simple, interpretable one near the prediction point (Ribeiro et al., 2016). In clinical settings, this might help explain why a patient was flagged as high risk for readmission, thereby supporting individualized care decisions. We focus on LIME in this chapter.

Another distinction is between *intrinsic* and *post-hoc* explainability. Intrinsic explainability is built into models like logistic regression and decision trees, which allow direct interpretation through their parameters and structures. Post-hoc methods, in contrast, are used to explain complex models that are not interpretable by default. Techniques such as global surrogates, SHAP, MAPLE, and local rule-based explanations fall into this category. These methods are critical in healthcare settings where complex models are often needed for high accuracy but still require interpretability to meet ethical and clinical standards.

Explainability methods can also be categorized as *model-agnostic* or *model-specific*. Model-agnostic tools—like LIME and SHAP—work with any model type, making them especially valuable for heterogeneous healthcare applications where multiple modeling approaches may be explored. Model-specific methods, such as attention mechanisms in deep learning or gain-based importance scores in decision trees, offer insights tailored to a specific algorithm. These techniques are generally more precise but lack the flexibility to generalize across model classes.

Lastly, a *stakeholder-centered* approach to explainability is crucial in healthcare. Clinicians, patients, regulators, and researchers each require different forms of interpretability. Clinicians seek explanations that fit into diagnostic reasoning; patients need understandable and trustworthy outputs; regulators demand clarity for accountability and safety; and researchers look for mechanisms to generate and test new hypotheses. From an organizational perspective, explainability also plays a key role in decision-making, trust-building, and regulatory compliance. Health management studies suggest that explainable AI enhances the dynamic capabilities of health organizations—enabling them to sense, learn, and integrate new technologies effectively (Leung, 2012). Additionally, legal frameworks such as the GDPR emphasize the "right to explanation" for individuals affected by automated decision-making (Goodman & Flaxman, 2017), further highlighting the need for well-structured interpretability in healthcare AI.

Using LIME for Local Interpretability

LIME (Local Interpretable Model-Agnostic Explanations) is a prominent technique designed to interpret individual predictions from complex, often opaque, machine learning models (Ribeiro et al., 2016). It operates by approximating the model's behavior in the vicinity of a specific data point using a simplified, interpretable model—typically a linear regression. This local approximation is achieved by perturbing the input features of the target instance, observing the corresponding changes in model predictions, and then fitting a weighted surrogate model to the perturbed dataset. The result is a local explanation that reveals the most influential features contributing to that particular prediction.

The theoretical innovation of LIME lies in its attention to the "locality" of explanations. Unlike global interpretability approaches that seek to understand the model as a whole, LIME acknowledges that a model's behavior may vary substantially across different regions of the feature space. By focusing on a small neighborhood around an individual instance, LIME allows analysts to capture highly non-linear behavior in a way that remains intelligible to humans. This focus on local fidelity makes LIME particularly well-suited for high-stakes domains like healthcare, where personalized predictions require clear justification.

LIME's methodology is underpinned by three key components. First, it constructs an *interpretable representation*, such as binary indicators that represent whether a feature value exceeds a threshold. Second, it performs *locality-aware sampling*, creating synthetic variations of the original instance and weighting them by their proximity in feature space. Third, it trains a *surrogate model*, usually linear, on the weighted samples to approximate the original model's behavior near the point of interest. These steps ensure that the explanation remains both faithful to the original model and understandable to a human analyst.

In healthcare settings, applying LIME requires special consideration. *Feature engineering* must account for clinical nuances, such as how comorbidities or physiological markers interact. *Clinical relevance* is essential in designing realistic perturbations—changes in laboratory results or demographic factors should reflect plausible medical scenarios. Finally, healthcare data often contain *temporal dependencies*, particularly in time-series records or longitudinal patient data. LIME's standard implementation may not capture these nuances without customization, suggesting that adaptations or alternative tools may be required for temporal explainability.

Steps to Use LIME in R

This section outlines how to apply LIME in RStudio using the simulated EHR dataset introduced in Chap. 8. Several steps are involved:

1. **Prepare the Data**
   Clean and preprocess the dataset by handling missing values and encoding categorical variables as needed for machine learning models.
2. **Train the Model**
   Build a complex model such as a random forest or gradient boosting model using the training data.
3. **Set Up the LIME Explainer**
   Configure the LIME explainer by specifying appropriate parameters, including the number of bins for numeric variables and the distance function used to assess similarity between data points.
4. **Generate Local Explanations**
   Use LIME to generate case-level explanations for model predictions. This is especially useful for examining high-risk cases or unusual outcomes.
5. **Validate with Clinical Experts**

Review the explanations with domain experts to confirm they are clinically valid and useful for interpretation in practice.

Worked Example: Simulated SUD Dataset

We now apply LIME to the simulated EHR dataset from Chap. 8 (see Fig. 9.1). This dataset contains features such as age, BMI, glucose levels, and family history of substance use disorder (SUD). For this example, we assume that a random forest model (`rf_model`) has already been trained using the training dataset (`train`). The testing dataset is referred to as `test`.

The R scripts, shown in Fig. 9.1, perform supervised machine learning to classify substance use disorder (SUD) status using a random forest model. It begins by ensuring that the required packages—`lime`, `caret`, `randomForest`, and `dplyr`—are installed and loaded into the R session. These packages are essential for model building, evaluation, and interpretation.

The next step involves preparing the training and testing datasets. The outcome variable `SUD_Status` is converted to a factor to ensure compatibility with

```r
# ---------------- Packages --------------------------------------------------
if (!requireNamespace("lime", quietly = TRUE)) install.packages("lime")
if (!requireNamespace("caret", quietly = TRUE)) install.packages("caret")
if (!requireNamespace("randomForest", quietly = TRUE)) install.packages("randomForest")
if (!requireNamespace("dplyr", quietly = TRUE)) install.packages("dplyr")

# ---------------- Load required packages ----------------
library(caret)
library(randomForest)
library(lime)
library(dplyr)
library(ggplot2)

# ---------------- Prepare the data ----------------
# Ensure target variable is a factor for classification
train$SUD_Status <- as.factor(train$SUD_Status)
test$SUD_Status  <- as.factor(test$SUD_Status)

# Split into predictors and outcome
train_x <- train %>% select(-SUD_Status)
train_y <- train$SUD_Status

# ---------------- Train the model using caret ----------------
set.seed(123)
rf_model2 <- train(
  x = train_x,
  y = train_y,
  method = "rf",
  ntree = 500,
  trControl = trainControl(method = "cv", number = 5)
)

```

Fig. 9.1 Data preprocessing steps for the Local Interpretable Model-Agnostic Explanations (LIME) procedures in RStudio

```r
# ---------------- Build LIME explainer -----------------------------------
explainer <- lime::lime(
  x              = train_x,        # predictor variables from training data
  model          = rf_model2,      # trained caret model
  bin_continuous = TRUE,           # discretize numeric variables
  n_bins         = 5,              # number of bins for binning
  quantile_bins  = TRUE            # use quantile-based binning
)

# ======================================================================
# 📊 Part 1: Generic feature importance from 100 test cases
# ======================================================================
set.seed(42)
sample_size <- 100  # number of cases to use for generic explanation
cases_x <- test %>%
  dplyr::slice_sample(n = sample_size) %>%
  dplyr::select(-SUD_Status)  # keep only predictor variables

# Generate LIME explanations for the sample
explanations <- lime::explain(
  x            = cases_x,
  explainer    = explainer,
  n_labels     = 1,                # explain the top predicted class
  n_features   = 8,                # number of features to include per case
  n_samples    = 5000,
  dist_fun     = "gower",
  kernel_width = 0.75
)
```

Fig. 9.2 Building the Local Interpretable Model-Agnostic Explanations (LIME) explainer and generating LIME explanations in RStudio

classification algorithms in R. The dataset is then split into predictor variables (`train_x`) and the target outcome (`train_y`). This separation allows the model to focus on learning the relationship between features and the classification label.

Following data preparation, the program fits a random forest model using the `method` = `"rf"` function. This function wraps around the random forest algorithm to streamline training and model validation. It then uses 500 trees (ntree = 500) and performs 5-fold cross-validation to assess model performance and reduce the risk of overfitting. A random seed is set for reproducibility, ensuring consistent results across different runs. The resulting model object (rf_model2) is ready for use in prediction, evaluation, or further interpretation using model explanation tools like LIME.

The R code depicted in Fig. 9.2 generates a **generic explanation** of variable importance using the LIME (Local Interpretable Model-agnostic Explanations) framework. This approach helps to understand which features are consistently influential in the model's predictions across multiple cases, rather than focusing on a single individual.

As shown in Fig. 9.2, the process begins by building a LIME explainer using the training data (train_x) and the previously trained random forest model (rf_model2).

```
# Aggregate feature importance
generic_importance <- explanations %>%
  dplyr::group_by(feature) %>%
  dplyr::summarise(mean_abs_weight = mean(abs(feature_weight))) %>%
  dplyr::arrange(desc(mean_abs_weight))

print(generic_importance)

# Plot aggregated importance
ggplot(generic_importance,
       aes(x = reorder(feature, mean_abs_weight),
           y = mean_abs_weight)) +
  geom_col(fill = "steelblue") +
  coord_flip() +
  labs(
    title = "Average Absolute LIME Feature Importance (n = 100 cases)",
    x = "Feature",
    y = "Average |Weight|"
  )
```

Fig. 9.3 R scripts to generate feature importance for the LIME explanations in RStudio

The LIME explainer is configured to bin continuous variables into five quantile-based intervals. This discretization simplifies the interpretation of continuous predictors by turning them into categorical-like bins, which LIME can handle more effectively when generating explanations.

Next, the code randomly selects 100 test observations from the test dataset. This sampling is done to create a representative subset of individuals for whom local explanations will be generated. Only the predictor variables are retained (select (-SUD_Status)) since the LIME algorithm focuses on explaining model outputs based on input features.

Once the sample is prepared, the lime::explain() function is called to generate local explanations for each case. For each observation, LIME produces a breakdown of how much each feature contributes to the predicted outcome, based on 5000 simulated data points and a Gower distance metric. It selects the top 8 contributing features per case and uses a kernel width of 0.75 to weight the simulated samples.

To obtain a general picture of feature importance, the code aggregates the results from all 100 local explanations. It calculates the mean of the absolute feature weights across all observations, which reflects the average influence of each feature regardless of direction (positive or negative). This summary is stored in the generic_importance data frame and sorted in descending order of importance. Figure 9.3 contains the R code to visualize the generic_importance object in RStudio. It uses the ggplot function to create a chart to display the importance of various feature variables:

The R code in Fig. 9.3 creates a horizontal bar chart. As shown in Fig. 9.4, the chart displays each feature on the y-axis and its average absolute weight on the x-axis, providing an interpretable summary of which variables most strongly

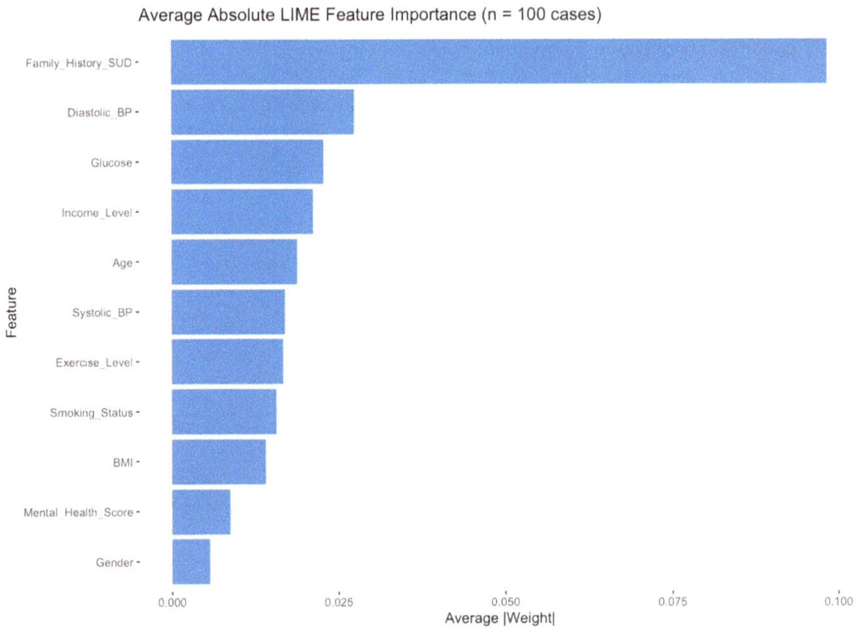

Fig. 9.4 A bar chart of generic feature importance in RStudio

influence the model's decisions across a range of cases. This output can be used to inform analysts, clinicians, or stakeholders about the relative significance of different predictors in the model (see Fig. 9.4):

LIME is a method designed to provide local explanations, meaning it focuses on how a predictive model arrives at its decision for a specific case rather than attempting to explain the entire model. This approach is useful when the goal is to understand the reasoning behind a single prediction, such as in clinical or operational decision-making.

The following R script and graph illustrate this local perspective. It shows the top features that contributed to the model's prediction for one test observation. Each bar represents how much a particular variable influenced the model's output, either positively or negatively. For example, if features such as age, glucose level, or family history strongly affected the predicted risk of substance use disorder for the selected individual, those variables will appear prominently in the plot.

By focusing on one case at a time, LIME makes complex models like random forests more interpretable. This supports the evaluation of individual decisions, helping users to validate and trust the model's recommendations in real-world settings.

The R script (see Fig. 9.5) focuses on a specific observation using the LIME model:

The graph (see Fig. 9.6) is generated in RStudio:

```r
# ===========================================================================
# 🔍 Part 2: Explain one specific observation
# ===========================================================================
# Select one high-risk case (SUD_Status == 1)
case_1_idx <- which(test$SUD_Status == 1)[1]
case_1_x <- test[case_1_idx, ] %>% select(-SUD_Status)

# Generate LIME explanation
explanation_1 <- lime::explain(
  x            = case_1_x,
  explainer    = explainer,
  n_labels     = 1,
  n_features   = 8,
  n_samples    = 5000,
  dist_fun     = "gower",
  kernel_width = 0.75
)

# Plot LIME explanation for one case
plot_features(explanation_1)

```

Fig. 9.5 R scripts to explain feature importance of one specific observation (e.g., a patient) in RStudio

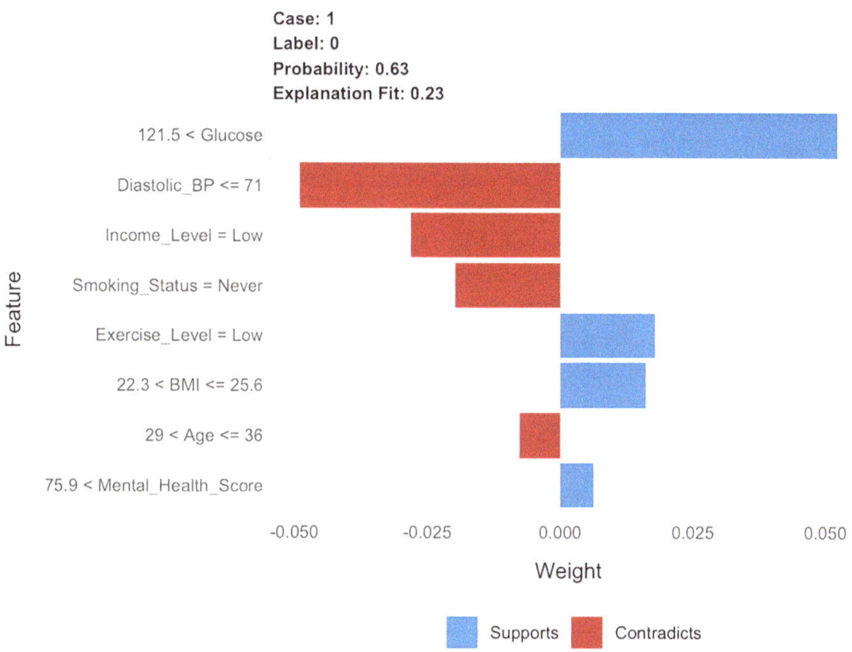

Fig. 9.6 A bar chart of feature importance for one observation (e.g., patient) in RStudio

```
103 # ======================================================================
104 # 🔍 Part 3: Explain six observations and visualize together
105 # ======================================================================
106 # Select six positive-class observations
107 case_6_idx <- which(test$SUD_Status == 1)[1:6]
108 cases_6_x <- test[case_6_idx, ] %>% select(-SUD_Status)
109
110 # Generate explanations for six cases
111 explanation_6 <- lime::explain(
112   x            = cases_6_x,
113   explainer    = explainer,
114   n_labels     = 1,
115   n_features   = 8,
116   n_samples    = 5000,
117   dist_fun     = "gower",
118   kernel_width = 0.75
119 )
120
121 # Plot all six explanations in one faceted plot (3 columns, automatic rows)
122 plot_features(
123   explanation_6,
124   ncol = 3
125 )
126
```

Fig. 9.7 R scripts to compare feature importance of six specific observations (e.g., six patients) in RStudio

While LIME is designed to explain model predictions at the individual level, analysts may also find it useful to compare explanations across **multiple cases**, particularly those with a common characteristic such as being classified as substance use disorder (SUD) patients. This comparative approach has practical value in identifying consistent patterns or distinguishing features across individuals in the same risk group.

The following graph presents LIME explanations for several test cases predicted as SUD-positive. Each subplot corresponds to one patient and highlights the top features that contributed to their individual prediction. By comparing these explanations side by side, the analyst can evaluate whether the model consistently relies on similar variables or adapts its reasoning for each case. The corresponding R script is shown in Fig. 9.7:

In Fig. 9.7, lines 121–125 of the R scripts are included to produce the graph in RStudio as shown in Fig. 9.8:

The graph in Fig. 9.8 shows how each factor affects the selected observations by illustrating the top features contributing to the model's predictions for each case. Such comparisons can support pattern recognition, guide follow-up investigations, and inform personalized interventions. For instance, if features like family history, glucose levels, and BMI consistently emerge as influential across multiple patients, these variables may warrant closer examination during clinical assessments or care planning. This type of analysis helps translate model output into actionable insights.

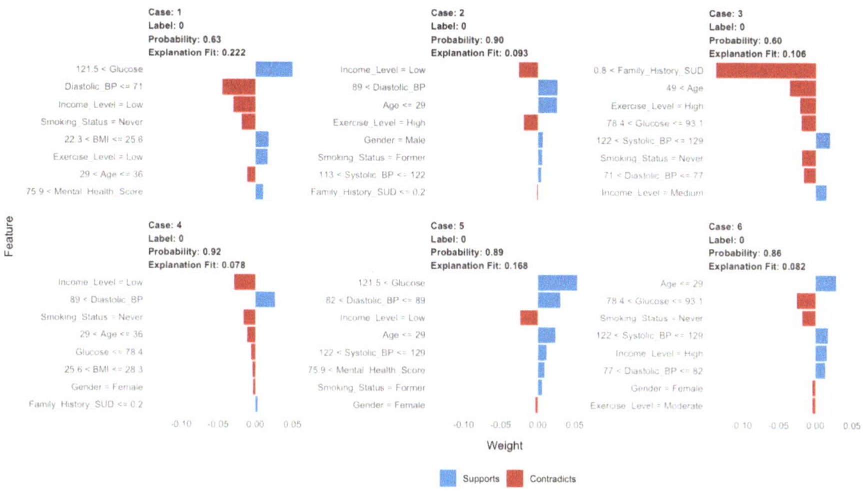

Fig. 9.8 Displaying feature importance for six observations (e.g., six patients) in RStudio

Limitations and Considerations

Explainability is a critical component in the responsible application of AI and machine learning in public health. While this chapter focuses primarily on technical explanations using tools like LIME, the broader goal of explainability is to increase trust, transparency, and accountability in AI-supported decisions. By making complex models more understandable, explainability empowers researchers, clinicians, and public health professionals to interpret and validate model outputs, identify potential biases, and ensure that AI tools align with clinical reasoning and ethical standards. In this way, explainability contributes to the "un-black-boxing" of machine learning systems, which is essential for gaining confidence in AI applications that may influence individual care or population-level policy.

LIME (Local Interpretable Model-agnostic Explanations) is one widely used method for improving model interpretability, especially in healthcare settings. However, it comes with several important limitations.

One major concern is instability. LIME relies on random sampling around the input instance to generate explanations, which can lead to slight variations in results between runs. In clinical environments where consistency and reproducibility are essential for trust and decision-making, this variability may limit LIME's practical utility unless properly controlled—for example, by setting a fixed random seed.

Another limitation involves feature correlation. LIME assumes independence among input variables when generating synthetic samples. Yet, many clinical variables, such as blood pressure, cholesterol, and BMI, are highly correlated. Ignoring these relationships can produce misleading or clinically implausible explanations, reducing the method's reliability in practice.

A third issue concerns surrogate model fidelity. LIME uses a simpler local model—typically linear regression—to approximate the predictions of a complex machine learning model in a small neighborhood of the input. If the true model behaves non-linearly even within this local region, the surrogate model may not capture important decision boundaries, leading to inaccurate or oversimplified interpretations.

Despite these limitations, LIME remains useful when applied carefully. Its visual outputs—such as bar plots showing the top contributing features for an individual prediction—enable users to ask, "Why did the model classify this patient as high risk?" and receive a reasoned explanation. When validated and aligned with clinical knowledge, LIME has been shown to increase user trust and support informed decision-making (Tonekaboni et al., 2019). However, successful implementation depends on ensuring that explanations are meaningful within the context of clinical practice.

As an alternative, SHAP (SHapley Additive exPlanations) provides a more theoretically grounded framework for interpretability (Lundberg & Lee, 2017). SHAP supports both local and global explanations and is based on cooperative game theory, attributing a model's prediction to individual features according to their marginal contributions. This method satisfies desirable properties such as efficiency, symmetry, and additivity, making it more stable and consistent than LIME across multiple observations. In healthcare, SHAP is often preferred because it enables both case-specific insight and broader pattern recognition across patient populations.

Reproducibility and Generative AI: A New Challenge

Generative AI tools such as ChatGPT are increasingly used in healthcare research for code generation, data simulation, and documentation. While these tools offer notable efficiency benefits, they also introduce new challenges related to reproducibility. Because models like ChatGPT are probabilistic and context-sensitive, identical prompts may yield different outputs across sessions or model versions. This variability poses a risk to scientific workflows, particularly in healthcare, where consistency is crucial for regulatory compliance and clinical validation.

These concerns compound existing reproducibility challenges in health-related machine learning, including restricted data access, software dependencies, and incomplete documentation (McDermott et al., 2021). Variability in AI-generated outputs can complicate replication and affect downstream analyses, such as automated modeling or synthetic dataset generation.

To mitigate these risks, researchers should implement safeguards such as setting random seeds, standardizing prompts, recording model versions, and combining AI-generated content with expert oversight. A more comprehensive discussion of reproducibility strategies—including technical, methodological, and organizational approaches—will be provided in Chap. 10.

Discussion Questions

1. What are the key benefits and limitations of LIME compared to SHAP in public health analytics? Consider both technical aspects and practical implementation challenges in healthcare settings.
2. How might reproducibility issues affect the use of ChatGPT in academic or clinical research, and what comprehensive mitigation strategies would you recommend beyond the basic practices discussed?
3. When might you prioritize interpretability over predictive performance in a public health setting? Provide specific examples and discuss the ethical implications of each choice.
4. What strategies would you propose to increase transparency when using black-box models in clinical decision-support systems? Consider both technical and organizational approaches.
5. How do regulatory requirements for AI explainability impact the choice of machine learning methods in healthcare applications? Discuss the implications for model development, validation, and deployment.
6. How might the dynamic capabilities framework apply to healthcare organizations implementing explainable AI systems? What sensing, learning, and integrating capabilities would be most critical?
7. What role should patients play in the development and evaluation of explainable AI systems in healthcare? How might patient perspectives on explanations differ from those of healthcare professionals?

References

Breiman, L. (2001). Random forests. *Machine Learning, 45*(1), 5–32. https://doi.org/10.1023/A:1010933404324

Doshi-Velez, F., & Kim, B. (2017). Towards a rigorous science of interpretable machine learning. *arXiv preprint*, arXiv:1702.08608. https://arxiv.org/abs/1702.08608

Goodman, B., & Flaxman, S. (2017). European Union regulations on algorithmic decision-making and a "right to explanation". *AI Magazine, 38*(3), 50–57. https://doi.org/10.1609/aimag.v38i3.2741

Holzinger, A., Biemann, C., Pattichis, C. S., & Kell, D. B. (2017). What do we need to build explainable AI systems for the medical domain? *arXiv preprint*, arXiv:1712.09923. https://arxiv.org/abs/1712.09923

Leung, R. (2012). Health information technology and dynamic capabilities. *Health Care Management Review, 37*(1), 63–74. https://doi.org/10.1097/HMR.0b013e31823c9b67

Lipton, Z. C. (2018). The mythos of model interpretability: In machine learning, the concept of interpretability is both important and slippery. *Queue, 16*(3), 31–57. https://doi.org/10.1145/3236386.3241340

Lundberg, S. M., & Lee, S. I. (2017). A unified approach to interpreting model predictions. In *Proceedings of the 31st international conference on neural information processing systems* (pp. 4765–4774) https://arxiv.org/abs/1705.07874

McDermott, M. B., Wang, S., Marinsek, N., Ranganath, R., Foschini, L., & Ghassemi, M. (2021). Reproducibility in machine learning for health research: Still a ways to go. *Science Translational Medicine, 13*(586), eabb1655. https://doi.org/10.1126/scitranslmed.abb1655

Ribeiro, M. T., Singh, S., & Guestrin, C. (2016). “Why should I trust you?”: Explaining the predictions of any classifier. In *Proceedings of the 22nd ACM SIGKDD international conference on knowledge discovery and data mining* (pp. 1135–1144) https://arxiv.org/abs/1602.04938

Tonekaboni, S., Joshi, S., McCradden, M. D., & Goldenberg, A. (2019). What clinicians want: Contextualizing explainable machine learning for clinical end use. In *Proceedings of the 4th machine learning for healthcare conference* (pp. 359–380) https://arxiv.org/abs/1905.05134

Chapter 10
Future Directions and Continuous Learning in AI

Learning Objectives

By the end of this chapter, students should be able to:

1. **Explain** the current role of generative AI (GenAI) in public health practice and education.
2. **Identify** the reproducibility challenges posed by large language models (LLMs).
3. **Assess** the ethical considerations and evolving frameworks necessary for the responsible use of AI.
4. **Describe** the components of effective AI literacy programs.
5. **Evaluate** future applications of AI and their potential risks and benefits.

Introduction

The integration of artificial intelligence (AI) into public health represents a major technological turning point in the evolution of public health and related fields. As we stand at this transformative juncture, public health professionals, educators, and researchers must critically examine how best to engage with generative AI (GenAI), especially large language models (LLMs), in ways that enhance scientific progress while upholding the rigor and ethics central to the field. This chapter analyzes the current landscape of AI use in public health, foregrounds emerging challenges such as reproducibility and responsible application, and explores the pedagogical and institutional shifts necessary to ensure meaningful integration.

The rapid proliferation of GenAI tools—ranging from general-purpose platforms like ChatGPT and Claude to domain-specific applications in clinical and epidemiological research—has reshaped public health methodologies. These tools are already

Supplementary Information The online version contains supplementary material available at https://doi.org/10.1007/978-3-032-08677-8_10.

R. Leung, *Leveraging GenAI for Machine Learning Education in Public Health*,
https://doi.org/10.1007/978-3-032-08677-8_10

influencing how we generate hypotheses, conduct analyses, design educational content, and formulate interventions. The urgency lies not in debating whether GenAI belongs in public health, but in developing frameworks for its responsible, ethical, and practical use. As with earlier technological revolutions, such as the introduction of statistical software and GIS, the challenge is to adapt our practices, not resist them.

The opportunities presented by GenAI are far-reaching, including accelerated research productivity, enhanced public health surveillance, and broader access to decision-support tools. Recent research demonstrates that AI can support public health surveillance, epidemiological research, communication, resource allocation, and other forms of decision-making, with the potential to revolutionize both practice and research (Panteli et al., 2025). At the same time, these benefits are accompanied by new forms of uncertainty—ranging from algorithmic bias and lack of transparency to concerns about data integrity and ethical misuse. Public health professionals must learn to navigate this evolving terrain by balancing innovation with caution, and by developing skills that enable critical engagement with AI-generated content.

The integration of AI in public health education and practice faces significant challenges that require careful consideration. As noted in recent scholarship, there are persistent concerns about maintaining public trust, ensuring health equity and ethical behavior, and implementing new technologies across the workforce, requiring partnerships across academic institutions, government, and community stakeholders (Bharel et al., 2024). These challenges underscore the importance of developing robust frameworks for responsible AI deployment in public health contexts.

This chapter aims to provide a structured overview of GenAI's current and potential impact on public health. It begins by examining the normalization of GenAI in public health education and practice, followed by a discussion of its limitations—especially with regard to reproducibility. It then addresses how pedagogical and ethical frameworks must evolve and concludes by exploring future scenarios for GenAI applications in research, operations, and education. Through this exploration, the chapter offers guidance for integrating GenAI into public health in a way that is scientifically robust, ethically grounded, and strategically forward-looking.

GenAI Is Present, Not Future

The Current Reality of AI Integration

Generative AI (GenAI), including tools such as ChatGPT, Claude, and specialized medical AI systems, is no longer a speculative technology of the future—it has become an integral part of the contemporary technological landscape. Recent surveys indicate that two in three physicians are using health AI (American Medical Association, 2025), with more than four out of ten medical groups (43%) reporting added or expanded use of AI in 2024 (Medical Group Management Association, 2024). Three-quarters of healthcare providers and pharmaceutical professionals believe artificial intelligence-related technologies will be "widespread" within the next 3 years. Even young children are being exposed to AI capabilities through educational platforms and consumer applications, suggesting that AI literacy will become as fundamental as digital literacy in the coming decades.

Despite the large number of professionals having experimented with AI tools, trust levels remain a concern. Those who said their concerns exceeded their enthusiasm for the technology dropped to 25% in 2024, down from 29% in 2023, while data privacy (72%) and ethical concerns remain significant barriers to adoption. This reflects that general apprehension toward AI is still prevalent among healthcare professionals, though attitudes are gradually shifting. Only 38% of Americans say AI being used to do things like diagnose disease and recommend treatments would lead to better health outcomes for patients generally, indicating that public trust in AI applications remains limited (Tyson et al., 2023).

Rather than attempting to ban or ignore GenAI, educators and public health professionals must actively learn how to use it effectively. The integration of AI into public health education and research is not merely a technological upgrade—it represents a fundamental shift in how we process information, generate hypotheses, and conduct research. This transformation parallels previous technological revolutions in public health, from the introduction of statistical software packages to the adoption of geographic information systems (GIS) for epidemiological surveillance.

AI's Transformative Potential in Public Health Education

In public health education and research, understanding both the strengths and limitations of GenAI is essential for maintaining scientific rigor while embracing technological innovation. The integration of AI within public health education shows transformative potential in crafting individualized educational programs, though comprehensive training remains essential. Incorporating AI into the development and delivery of public health curricula represents a revolutionary step, providing a dynamic and responsive educational model. As Wang and Li (2024) emphasize, AI-enhanced learning environments significantly improve hypothesis generation and research efficiency when paired with critical thinking and methodological training.

GenAI's usefulness lies in its ability to synthesize large volumes of information and respond to a wide range of prompts quickly. This capability makes it a powerful tool for learning, brainstorming, and creating initial drafts of scientific writing or coding. For example, AI can help public health researchers quickly identify relevant literature, generate code for statistical analyses, or draft sections of grant proposals. However, the use of GenAI should be accompanied by comprehensive training and oversight to ensure quality, accuracy, and ethical use.

Institutional Adaptation and AI Literacy

Those who choose not to engage with these technologies risk falling behind, as AI-supported practices become increasingly normalized in both academic and professional settings. As GenAI technologies are integrated more deeply into academic and research settings, establishing clear definitions and strategies around AI literacy becomes essential. Georgiva et al. (2024) propose a durable framework for AI Literacy in Teaching and Learning (ALTL) that emphasizes the practical, ethical, and institutional dimensions of AI use in higher education. Yet, a significant skills gap remains, with only 24% of respondents in one survey reporting AI training from their employers.

The challenge for educational institutions is not simply to teach students how to use AI tools, but to help them develop the critical thinking skills necessary to evaluate AI outputs and integrate them appropriately into their work. This requires a fundamental rethinking of pedagogical approaches, moving from information transmission models to more collaborative, inquiry-based learning that emphasizes critical evaluation and synthesis. Effective AI literacy requires not only practical application—through the integration of AI tools in teaching, research, and administration—but also careful attention to ethics (Long & Magerko 2020). As Long and Magerko (2020) argued, AI literacy must combine technical skills and critical reflection to ensure individuals can responsibly and effectively engage with AI technologies.

For example, most graduate programs have courses on research methods, quantitative and/or qualitative methodology. Having a course on GenAI may become standard in the future as faculty can safely assume that many students will use GenAI tools such as ChatGPT, so one or more courses to teach how these tools can be properly used may become the norm and would be useful for future public health professionals and faculty. It is necessary for policymakers to integrate AI literacy into curricular standards, working together with subject matter experts and educators to define age-appropriate AI literacy competencies and integrate them into the curriculum (Yang et al., 2025).

Reproducibility and the Limits of AI

The aforementioned course or a general awareness among public health professionals is to understand that AI actually has several important setbacks. In the following, we look at reproducibility and related challenges that must be addressed for responsible AI integration in public health research.

The Reproducibility Crisis in AI-Assisted Research

A key step in responsibly integrating AI into public health research involves acknowledging its limitations, especially concerning reproducibility. While courses on GenAI and general awareness among public health professionals help demystify its functions, they must also emphasize the constraints that GenAI introduces into scientific workflows. Chief among these is the challenge of reproducing results—a fundamental principle of scientific validity. This section addresses reproducibility concerns in GenAI-assisted research, explores nuanced perspectives on what reproducibility should mean in the AI era, and outlines necessary frameworks and institutional responses.

Despite its transformative potential, GenAI—particularly large language models (LLMs)—raises significant concerns about reproducibility. LLMs like ChatGPT operate probabilistically: identical prompts can yield different responses across sessions depending on model version, temperature settings, and random seed values. This variability undermines consistency and makes replication of outputs difficult, violating a core standard of scientific rigor. As Baker (2024) notes, researchers have expressed alarm that the careless use of GenAI is contributing to an influx of irreproducible or unsubstantiated research. AI researchers themselves struggle to reproduce key results, which creates credibility risks for the scientific community at large.

This issue is especially acute in public health, where scientific findings often inform policy and clinical decision-making. Traditional research methods, though not immune to error, typically offer more controlled pathways to replication. In contrast, the integration of GenAI into research demands new strategies for documentation, version control, and workflow transparency. Moreover, as Kelly et al. (2019) highlight, machine learning (ML) applications in healthcare pose unique reproducibility challenges due to model complexity, shifting data environments, and inconsistent standards for evaluation. Addressing these issues is essential to ensure that AI methods produce findings that are both credible and safe for public health deployment.

Contextualizing Reproducibility in the AI Era

However, not all concerns about reproducibility should lead to rejection of GenAI tools. A more constructive approach is to reframe GenAI as an assistive rather than definitive tool in scientific workflows. For example, this book uses ChatGPT to aid R programming for machine learning applications. While GenAI-generated code snippets may differ slightly with each session, the finalized R scripts derived from them—especially when guided by techniques such as `set.seed()`—can achieve high reproducibility. In this way, GenAI functions as a support mechanism in the early, generative stages of research, after which researchers apply traditional coding and validation methods to ensure consistency.

Moreover, some reproducibility concerns that were valid in the pre-AI era may require reevaluation. Literature searches, for instance, are inherently dynamic—each search may retrieve new studies depending on the timing and platform used. Similarly, LLMs that scan ever-growing corpora will naturally yield evolving outputs. To address this, researchers using GenAI should document not only the content generated but also the prompts used, the time and context of generation, and any human modifications. While this transparency may not eliminate variability, it enables traceability and offers a more nuanced standard of reproducibility aligned with AI-era practices.

Balancing Innovation with Scientific Rigor

Integrating GenAI into public health research requires careful trade-offs between the benefits of automation and the need for scientific credibility. GenAI allows researchers to process and synthesize vast datasets that would otherwise be inaccessible for manual analysis, potentially uncovering novel patterns or hypotheses. Yet, these outputs must be verified through traditional empirical validation and peer-reviewed methods. Desai et al. (2025) stress that the reproducibility crisis in AI is exacerbated by confusion about validation protocols and an urgent need for clear evaluative standards.

A robust reproducibility framework must include structured documentation of AI interactions (such as prompt logs), model version control, and verification of AI-generated outputs. This also calls for educational interventions that teach researchers how to interpret GenAI outputs with a critical lens and validate results through conventional techniques. In public health, where research translates quickly into practice, this dual emphasis on innovation and rigor is especially vital.

Developing New Standards for AI-Assisted Research

To address these concerns systematically, professional organizations and research institutions must establish new norms for AI use. Transparency, validation, and ethical oversight must be foundational components. The American Public Health Association and similar institutions are beginning to issue guidance on AI in research settings, outlining core principles such as privacy, equity, safety, robustness, and accountability (APHA, 2025). However, these principles often remain aspirational in the absence of specific implementation tools and oversight mechanisms.

Creating enforceable standards for GenAI-assisted research requires interdisciplinary collaboration between technologists, public health experts, and research methodologists. Clear, shared protocols can help ensure that AI is used responsibly across diverse contexts. Public health organizations should also invest in modern data infrastructure, address workforce gaps in AI competency, and develop governance structures to monitor compliance. Ultimately, fostering a reproducible and trustworthy research environment depends not only on new technology but on institutional commitment to uphold the scientific values that define public health.

Responsible Use of AI: Rethinking Pedagogy and Ethics

The previous section outlined the technical and procedural challenges posed by GenAI, particularly the issue of reproducibility. However, addressing reproducibility alone is insufficient for responsible AI integration in public health. A broader and equally critical dimension involves rethinking the ethical and pedagogical frameworks that guide how AI is developed, implemented, and taught. As GenAI reshapes scientific processes, it also demands a reevaluation of the values, practices, and assumptions that underlie education and professional conduct in public health.

Evolving Ethical Frameworks for AI in Public Health

Responsible AI use goes beyond ensuring technical validity or minimizing algorithmic bias; it requires engagement with deeper ethical questions about the role of technology in shaping knowledge, practice, and equity. Traditional principles in public health ethics—beneficence, non-maleficence, autonomy, and justice—remain relevant but are insufficient on their own to address the sociotechnical complexity of AI. GenAI tools can reinforce systemic inequities if not critically assessed, particularly when used in data-driven decision-making about vulnerable populations.

Whittlestone et al. (2019) argue that AI ethics in public health must consider both short-term impacts and long-term societal consequences. Their framework emphasizes transparency in algorithm design, accountability for decision-making processes, and sustained engagement with affected communities. This perspective recognizes that AI systems are not neutral tools; they are embedded within social, political, and institutional structures that can either reinforce or challenge existing health disparities. As such, responsible AI use requires ethical foresight, interdisciplinary collaboration, and proactive governance.

Pedagogical Transformation in the AI Era

These ethical considerations must be integrated into educational practice. Just as reproducibility requires technical infrastructure and training, ethical AI use demands a pedagogical transformation that equips students to critically engage with AI technologies. Some educators express concern that GenAI tools erode foundational skills, such as critical thinking or methodological precision. However, historical patterns suggest otherwise. Technological innovations—from calculators to search engines—have often changed how we teach and learn, but they have not eliminated the importance of core competencies.

The imperative is not to resist change but to shape it thoughtfully. Public health educators should incorporate GenAI into classrooms in ways that reinforce rather than replace analytical reasoning and scientific rigor. Students should be taught how to use GenAI as a supplementary tool while maintaining academic integrity, curiosity, and methodological soundness. Critical evaluation of AI-generated content, recognition of model limitations, and awareness of context-specific risks must become standard components of public health education.

Developing AI Literacy Programs

To support this shift, institutions must design comprehensive AI literacy programs that address both technical fluency and ethical reasoning. These programs should teach students how AI systems function, how they produce outputs, and where they are most—and least—appropriate to use. Equally important is instruction on prompt engineering, the identification of hallucinated or biased outputs, and frameworks for interpreting AI-generated results within broader scientific and ethical contexts.

Kumar et al. (2025) provide a model for such a curriculum, incorporating modules on the mechanics of AI, ethical principles, practical applications, and critical evaluation strategies. Their findings show that students trained under this model demonstrated improved competency in using GenAI tools while upholding high standards of academic and scientific integrity. Such programs not only close skills gaps but also foster a new generation of professionals equipped to use AI responsibly and effectively in public health settings.

Technical and Ethical Evaluation Frameworks

As public health education evolves to promote AI literacy and ethical engagement, equal attention must be given to evaluating the performance and risks of GenAI systems in practice. Educators may prepare students to use GenAI responsibly, but those tools must also be subject to ongoing technical scrutiny and ethical oversight to ensure safe and effective use in real-world applications. Developing appropriate evaluation frameworks is therefore a critical next step in aligning AI innovation with public health values.

Understanding AI Limitations in Public Health Contexts

From a technical standpoint, GenAI models present several known limitations that carry significant implications for public health. One of the most concerning is the phenomenon of hallucination—when the model generates plausible-sounding but factually incorrect or entirely fabricated information. In public health and medicine, where information guides interventions, policy, and care delivery, such inaccuracies can have serious consequences. The danger is amplified by the credibility of AI-generated language, which may obscure the line between accurate insight and misinformation, particularly for users lacking domain expertise.

Bias is another persistent concern. GenAI models trained on large-scale data inherit the social, cultural, and institutional biases embedded in that data. When deployed in public health contexts, these models can reinforce or even amplify disparities rooted in systemic inequities. Without robust evaluation, AI tools may unintentionally propagate unequal treatment, misrepresent population-level trends, or guide resource allocation in ways that disadvantage historically marginalized communities.

Developing Comprehensive Evaluation Frameworks

To mitigate these risks, GenAI systems used in public health must be assessed through structured, multidimensional frameworks. Evaluation should include technical performance metrics—such as accuracy, consistency, and reliability—but must also go further to assess ethical alignment, safety, and social implications. Ma et al. (2025) propose a comprehensive model that evaluates GenAI tools across several dimensions: bias detection, safety impact, usability, and ethical compliance. Such frameworks offer a systematic way to assess whether AI tools meet the demands of both scientific rigor and social responsibility.

These evaluation processes must be collaborative by design. Responsible deployment of GenAI in public health requires partnerships among data scientists, health researchers, educators, ethicists, and regulators. No single discipline can fully anticipate the consequences of AI use in complex public systems. Therefore, inclusive and cross-sectoral collaboration is essential to ensure that evaluation frameworks are rigorous, implementable, and contextually relevant across diverse populations and settings.

Implementing Quality Assurance Measures

Beyond general frameworks, quality assurance (QA) procedures tailored to specific use cases are essential to ensure that AI tools function safely and as intended. In research settings, QA might include peer-reviewed validation of AI-generated analyses, clear documentation of AI usage, and replication of key findings using traditional methods. For clinical applications, QA protocols could involve real-time human oversight, decision auditing, and systematic monitoring of AI outputs for reliability and fairness.

The development and maintenance of these "AI-QA" measures should be supported by institutional and regulatory infrastructure. Professional organizations and public health agencies must play a proactive role in defining and enforcing standards for AI use. These standards must be dynamic—able to evolve as new AI capabilities emerge—while maintaining transparency, accountability, and alignment with public health goals. Ultimately, the success of GenAI in public health will depend not only on its technical sophistication but on our collective ability to govern it responsibly.

Future Scenarios and Expansion of GenAI in Public Health

Having considered the technical and ethical responsibilities associated with GenAI use in public health, it is important to turn toward the horizon. As frameworks for evaluation and quality assurance are developed and institutionalized, they will serve as a foundation for expanding GenAI into a wider array of applications. While this book has focused on using GenAI to support machine learning programming in R for public health education and research, the potential reach of these technologies is significantly broader. With appropriate safeguards in place, GenAI is poised to transform many aspects of public health operations, policy, and care delivery.

Emerging Applications and Opportunities

Future applications of GenAI in public health extend across multiple domains. These include drug and vaccine development, disease detection and diagnosis, real-time surveillance systems, workforce forecasting, mental health screening, and operational optimization within healthcare systems. As technical performance improves and institutional capacity for responsible oversight increases, GenAI will likely become a standard tool in many of these areas.

In pharmaceutical research, for instance, GenAI tools are already being used to identify candidate therapeutic compounds, predict adverse drug interactions, and optimize clinical trial design. Companies such as DeepMind and BioNTech have demonstrated how AI can dramatically accelerate the drug discovery pipeline, reducing time and cost while enhancing precision (Aggarwal et al., 2025). As these tools become more sophisticated and transparent, their role in public health-oriented drug development will likely grow.

Transforming Public Health Surveillance

One of the most promising areas of GenAI application is real-time public health surveillance. By analyzing large, heterogeneous data sources—including social media content, electronic health records, environmental sensor data, and mobile health feeds—AI-powered systems can detect early warning signs of disease outbreaks and emerging health threats. These capabilities have the potential to supplement or even outperform traditional surveillance systems in speed and scope.

For example, Sadilek at al. (2018) describe an AI-powered platform that used aggregated web-search and location data to identify venues at elevated risk of foodborne illness in real time. Rather than relying solely on conventional complaint-based or routine inspections, the system leveraged machine learning to infer when a restaurant visit was followed by searches indicative of food poisoning. In deployments across two major U.S. cities, restaurants flagged by the model were over three times as likely to have serious health-code violations than venues selected by standard methods.

Workforce Development and Mental Health Applications

In addition to surveillance and diagnostics, GenAI also holds potential for addressing long-standing systemic challenges in workforce planning and mental health care. In workforce development, AI systems can analyze trends in labor markets, training pipelines, and demographic shifts to forecast future health workforce needs. These insights can inform policy decisions related to education, recruitment, and retention, helping to ensure a stable and responsive public health workforce.

In mental health, GenAI tools are increasingly used for screening and early intervention. AI-driven applications can identify individuals at risk of psychological distress by analyzing language patterns, social media behavior, or responses to self-assessment tools. When paired with appropriate referral and support systems, these tools can help expand access to mental health services and reduce the burden on overextended healthcare providers. However, as emphasized in earlier sections, any use of AI in such sensitive domains must be accompanied by rigorous ethical oversight and stakeholder engagement to prevent harm and ensure equitable implementation.

Conclusion: Shaping an Ethical Future for AI in Public Health

In summary, the challenge facing public health is not whether to adopt generative AI, but how to do so in a thoughtful, ethical, and scientifically grounded manner. As GenAI tools such as ChatGPT become increasingly embedded in academic, clinical, and policy environments, public health professionals must cultivate the knowledge and institutional infrastructure required to engage with these technologies responsibly. Understanding the strengths of GenAI—such as its capacity to synthesize information, automate routine tasks, and accelerate discovery—is essential. Equally important is recognizing its limitations, particularly in areas like reproducibility, bias, and misinformation. The future of GenAI in public health depends on our ability to balance innovation with oversight, speed with scrutiny, and opportunity with accountability.

This book seeks to make a practical contribution to that effort by focusing on a specific, accessible use case: using ChatGPT to support R programming for machine learning in public health contexts. By integrating GenAI into the process of learning coding and statistical modeling, the book offers a concrete pathway for students, educators, and researchers to build technical capacity while remaining aware of the broader implications of AI use. This applied focus serves a dual purpose: it enhances methodological skills while also providing a foundation for understanding how GenAI can—and should—be incorporated into scientific practice.

Looking ahead, future volumes may expand this approach by exploring how ChatGPT and other large language model (LLM) tools can assist with other dimensions of public health research and education. These may include literature review automation, public health communication, curriculum development, and policy simulation. Moreover, as AI technologies evolve, there is an opportunity to consider their use beyond public health, in fields such as environmental science, education, behavioral economics, and social justice. The responsible application of GenAI across disciplines will require interdisciplinary collaboration, continued ethical reflection, and adaptive learning structures that equip professionals to respond to rapid technological change.

Ultimately, shaping an ethical future for AI in public health is a collective task—one that requires engagement from researchers, educators, practitioners, students, and communities. By embedding principles of transparency, inclusivity, and scientific rigor into AI development and application, the public health field can ensure that technological innovation contributes meaningfully to health equity, population well-being, and sustainable systems of care.

Discussion Questions

1. In what ways is GenAI transforming traditional pedagogical and research practices in public health? How should public health programs adapt their curricula in response?

2. How do the probabilistic outputs of LLMs complicate the issue of reproducibility in scientific research? What steps can researchers take to mitigate these challenges?
3. Should the ethical frameworks in public health be revised in response to the rise of AI technologies? If so, what new elements should be included?
4. What are the key components of a responsible AI literacy program for public health students, and how do they address both technical and ethical dimensions?
5. Consider a future scenario in which AI is used for mental health screening in underserved communities. What safeguards would you propose to ensure ethical, equitable, and effective implementation?

References

Aggarwal, A., Banik, A., & Jha, V. K. (2025). Advances in pharmaceutical and rehabilitation sciences: From phytomedicine and nanotechnology to artificial intelligence in drug development and therapeutic management.

American Medical Association. (2025, February 26). 2 in 3 physicians are using health AI—up 78% from 2023. https://www.ama-assn.org/practice-management/digital-health/2-3-physicians-are-using-health-ai-78-2023

American Public Health Association. (2025). Equitably applying artificial intelligence in the United States workforce using training and collaboration. *NEW SOLUTIONS: A Journal of Environmental and Occupational Health Policy, 35*(2), 246–254. https://journals.sagepub.com/doi/abs/10.1177/10482911251337448

Baker, P. (2024). *Generative AI for dummies*. John Wiley & Sons. https://www.wiley.com/en-us/Generative+AI+For+Dummies-p-9781394270750.

Bharel, M., Auerbach, J., Nguyen, V., & DeSalvo, K. B. (2024). Transforming public health practice with generative artificial intelligence: Article examines how generative artificial intelligence could be used to transform public health practice in the US. *Health Affairs, 43*(6), 776–782.

Desai, A., Abdelhamid, M., & Padalkar, N. R. (2025). What is reproducibility in artificial intelligence and machine learning research? *AI Magazine, 46*(2), e70004. https://onlinelibrary.wiley.com/doi/full/10.1002/aaai.70004

Georgiva, M., Kassorla, M., & Papini, A. (2024). *AI literacy in teaching and learning: A durable framework for higher education*. Bipartisan Policy Center. https://bipartisanpolicy.org/blog/growing-need-for-ai-literacy/

Kelly, C. J., Karthikesalingam, A., Suleyman, M., Corrado, G., & King, D. (2019). Key challenges for delivering clinical impact with artificial intelligence. *BMC Medicine, 17*(1), 195. https://link.springer.com/article/10.1186/s12916-019-1426-2

Kumar, R., Singh, A., Kassar, A. S. A., Humaida, M. I., Joshi, S., & Sharma, M. (2025). Adoption challenges to artificial intelligence literacy in public healthcare: An evidence-based study in Saudi Arabia. *Frontiers in Public Health, 13*, 1558772. https://doi.org/10.3389/fpubh.2025.1558772

Long, D., & Magerko, B. (2020). What is AI literacy? Competencies and design considerations. In *Proceedings of the 2020 CHI conference on human factors in computing systems* (pp. 1–16). Association for Computing Machinery. https://doi.org/10.1145/3313831.3376727

Ma, X., Jiang, F., & Fang, X. (2025). Developing and evaluating an intelligent integration system for elderly care and health based on the sport-medicine-tourism model. *Frontiers in Public Health, 13*, 1523893. https://doi.org/10.3389/fpubh.2025.1523893

Medical Group Management Association. (2024). Pace of AI adoption in medical groups quickens in 2024. https://www.mgma.com/mgma-stat/pace-of-ai-adoption-in-medical-groups-quickens-in-2024

Panteli, D., Adib, K., Buttigieg, S., Goiana-da-Silva, F., Ladewig, K., Azzopardi-Muscat, N., et al. (2025). Artificial intelligence in public health: Promises, challenges, and an agenda for policy makers and public health institutions. *The Lancet Public Health, 10*(5), e428–e432.

Sadilek, A., Caty, S., DiPrete, L., Mansour, R., Schenk, T., Jr., Bergtholdt, M., et al. (2018). Machine-learned epidemiology: Real-time detection of foodborne illness at scale. *npj Digital Medicine, 1*(1), 36. https://www.nature.com/articles/s41746-018-0045-1

Tyson, A., Pasquini, G., Spencer, A., & Funk, C. (2023, February 22). 60% of Americans would be uncomfortable with provider relying on AI in their own health care: Yet many see promise for artificial intelligence to help issues of bias in medical care. Pew Research Center. https://www.pewresearch.org/science/2023/02/22/60-of-americans-would-be-uncomfortable-with-provider-relying-on-

Wang, J., & Li, J. (2024). Artificial intelligence empowering public health education: Prospects and challenges. *Frontiers in Public Health, 12*, 1389026. https://www.frontiersin.org/articles/10.3389/fpubh.2024.1389026/full

Whittlestone, J., Nyrup, R., Alexandrova, A., Dihal, K., & Cave, S. (2019). *Ethical and societal implications of algorithms, data, and artificial intelligence: A roadmap for research*. Nuffield Foundation, 1–59. https://www.nuffieldfoundation.org/wp-content/uploads/2019/02/Ethical-and-Societal-Implications-of-Data-and-AI-report-Nuffield-Foundat.pdf

Yang, Y., Zhang, Y., Sun, D., et al. (2025). Navigating the landscape of AI literacy education: Insights from a decade of research (2014–2024). *Humanities and Social Sciences Communications, 12*, 374. https://doi.org/10.1057/s41599-025-04583-8

Appendix: R/RStudio Scripts

Chapter 3

```
# Install caret package
install.packages("caret")

# Load the caret library
library(caret)

# Basic Arithmetic Operations
# Addition
5 + 3

# Subtraction
10 - 4

# Multiplication
6 * 7

# Division
20 / 5

# Exponentiation
2 ^ 3

# Assigning Variables
x <- 10
```

(continued)

R. Leung, *Leveraging GenAI for Machine Learning Education in Public Health*,
https://doi.org/10.1007/978-3-032-08677-8

Chapter 3 (continued)

```
y <- 5
z <- x + y
print(z)

# Creating a Vector
numbers <- c(1, 2, 3, 4, 5)
print(numbers)

# Loading the iris Dataset
data(iris)

# View the first few rows
head(iris)

# Check the structure
str(iris)

# Loading the BreastCancer Dataset
install.packages("mlbench")
# Load the package
library(mlbench)

# Load the dataset
data(BreastCancer)

# View the first few rows
head(BreastCancer)

# Check the structure
str(BreastCancer)

# Read an external dataset

# Step 1: Install the readr package
install.packages("readr")

# Step 2: Load the package
library(readr)

# Step 3: Set your working directory
```

(continued)

Chapter 3 (continued)

```
# Step 4: Read the CSV file
ehr_data <- read_csv("simulated_ehr_data_small.csv")

# Step 5: View the first few rows
head(ehr_data)

# Step 6: Check the structure of the dataset
str(ehr_data)

# Load ggplot2
library(ggplot2)

ggplot(ehr_data, aes(x = BMI)) +
 geom_histogram(binwidth = 2, fill = "steelblue", color = "black")
+
 theme_minimal() +
 labs(
  title = "Distribution of BMI in the Simulated EHR Dataset",
  x = "BMI",
  y = "Frequency"
 )
```

Chapter 4

```
data(iris)
install.packages("caret")
library("caret")
set.seed(123)
trainIndex <- createDataPartition(iris$Species, p = 0.8, list =
FALSE)
train_data <- iris[trainIndex, ]
test_data <- iris[-trainIndex, ]

# ==================================
===========================
# KNN with Iris Data Example
# ===================================
==========================
```

(continued)

Chapter 4 (continued)

```
# Load necessary packages
library(caret)
library(class)

# Load dataset
data(iris)

# Set random seed for reproducibility
set.seed(123)

# Split into training (80%) and test (20%) sets
trainIndex <- createDataPartition(iris$Species, p = 0.8, list =
FALSE)
train_data <- iris[trainIndex, ]
test_data  <- iris[-trainIndex, ]

# Normalize predictor variables
preProcValues <- preProcess(train_data[, 1:4], method = c
("center", "scale"))
train_data_norm <- predict(preProcValues, train_data[, 1:4])
test_data_norm <-  predict(preProcValues, test_data[, 1:4])

# Apply KNN (k = 5)
knn_predictions <- knn(train = train_data_norm,
             test = test_data_norm,
             cl = train_data$Species, k = 5)

# Evaluate accuracy
conf_matrix <- confusionMatrix(knn_predictions,
test_data$Species)
print(conf_matrix)

# ==========================================
======================
# Logistic Regression with mtcars Data Example
# ==========================================
======================
```

(continued)

Chapter 4 (continued)

```
# Load necessary libraries
library(caret)
library(dplyr)

# Load the dataset
data(mtcars)

# Convert outcome variable to factor (am: 0 = automatic, 1 = manual)
mtcars$am <- as.factor(mtcars$am)

# Set seed for reproducibility
set.seed(123)

# Split data into training (80%) and testing (20%)
trainIndex <- createDataPartition(mtcars$am, p = 0.8, list =
FALSE)
train_data <- mtcars[trainIndex, ]
test_data  <- mtcars[-trainIndex, ]

# Fit logistic regression model
logit_model <- glm(am ~ mpg + hp + wt, data = train_data, family =
binomial)

# Summary of model
summary(logit_model)

# Predict probabilities on test data
pred_probs <- predict(logit_model, newdata = test_data, type =
"response")

# Convert probabilities to binary class (threshold = 0.5)
pred_class <- ifelse(pred_probs > 0.5, 1, 0)
pred_class <- as.factor(pred_class)

# Confusion matrix
conf_matrix <- confusionMatrix(pred_class, test_data$am)
print(conf_matrix)

# ====================================
===========================
```

(continued)

Chapter 4 (continued)

```
# Decision Tree with titanic Data Example
# ================================
================================

# Install and load packages if needed
# install.packages("titanic")
library(titanic)
library(rpart)      # for decision tree
library(rpart.plot) # for plotting
library(caret)      # for train/test split and evaluation
library(dplyr)

# Prepare dataset (select relevant columns and remove NAs)
titanic_data <- titanic_train %>%
 select(Survived, Pclass, Sex, Age, SibSp, Parch, Fare, Embarked)
%>%
 na.omit()

# Convert variables to factors where appropriate
titanic_data$Survived <- as.factor(titanic_data$Survived)
titanic_data$Pclass   <- as.factor(titanic_data$Pclass)
titanic_data$Sex      <- as.factor(titanic_data$Sex)
titanic_data$Embarked <- as.factor(titanic_data$Embarked)

# Split into training and testing sets (80/20)
set.seed(123)
trainIndex <- createDataPartition(titanic_data$Survived, p =
0.8, list = FALSE)
train_data <- titanic_data[trainIndex, ]
test_data  <- titanic_data[-trainIndex, ]

# Ensure Survived in test_data has the same factor levels as in
train_data
test_data$Survived <- factor(test_data$Survived, levels = levels
(train_data$Survived))

# Fit decision tree model
tree_model <- rpart(Survived ~ Pclass + Sex + Age, data =
train_data, method = "class")
```

(continued)

Chapter 4 (continued)

```
# Visualize the decision tree
rpart.plot(tree_model)

# Predict on test data
tree_preds <- predict(tree_model, test_data, type = "class")

# Ensure predictions are factors with same levels as reference
tree_preds <- factor(tree_preds, levels = levels
(test_data$Survived))

# Confusion matrix
confusionMatrix(tree_preds, test_data$Survived)

# ==========================
===========================
# Decision Tree with titanic Data Example
# ===============================
=======================
# Load package
library(randomForest)
library(caret) # for confusionMatrix

# Fit Random Forest model
rf_model <- randomForest(
 Survived ~ Pclass + Sex + Age,
 data = train_data,    # assumes train_data already prepared
 ntree = 500,
 mtry = 2,
 importance = TRUE
)

# Predict on test data
rf_preds <- predict(rf_model, newdata = test_data, type =
"class")

# Confusion matrix
confusionMatrix(rf_preds, test_data$Survived)
```

Chapter 5

```
# Load caret
library(caret)

# Example: Use built-in mtcars dataset
data(mtcars)

# Set seed for reproducibility
set.seed(123)

# Create training (70%) and testing (30%) index
trainIndex <- createDataPartition(mtcars$mpg, p = 0.7, list =
FALSE)

# Split the data
train_data <- mtcars[trainIndex, ]
test_data  <- mtcars[-trainIndex, ]

# Linear regression on mtcars: fit, interpret, evaluate
library(caret)

# Load the data
data(mtcars)

# Set random seed for reproducibility
set.seed(123)

# Split data: 80% training, 20% testing
trainIndex <- createDataPartition(mtcars$mpg, p = 0.8, list =
FALSE)
train_data <- mtcars[trainIndex, ]
test_data  <- mtcars[-trainIndex, ]

# Fit linear regression model on training data
lm_model <- lm(mpg ~ wt + hp + cyl, data = train_data)

# View summary of the model
summary(lm_model)

# Predictions on the test set
pred_mpg <- predict(lm_model, newdata = test_data)
```

(continued)

Chapter 5 (continued)

```
# Evaluate model performance
mse <- mean((test_data$mpg - pred_mpg)^2)
rmse <- sqrt(mse)
rsq <- 1 - sum((test_data$mpg - pred_mpg)^2) / sum((test_data$mpg -
mean(test_data$mpg))^2)

# Print evaluation metrics
print(paste("Test MSE:", round(mse, 2)))
print(paste("Test RMSE:", round(rmse, 2)))
print(paste("Test R-squared:", round(rsq, 2)))

# 1) Load package
library(caret)

# 2) Load data
data(mtcars)

# 3) Reproducibility
set.seed(123)

# 4) Train/test split (80/20)
trainIndex <- createDataPartition(mtcars$mpg, p = 0.8, list =
FALSE)
train_data <- mtcars[trainIndex, ]
test_data  <- mtcars[-trainIndex, ]

# 5) Fit polynomial regression with wt^2 (raw quadratic term)
poly_model <- lm(mpg ~ wt + I(wt^2), data = train_data)

# 6) Model summary
summary(poly_model)

# 7) Predictions on test set
pred_mpg <- predict(poly_model, newdata = test_data)

# 8) Evaluation metrics: MSE, RMSE, R-squared
mse  <- mean((test_data$mpg - pred_mpg)^2)
rmse <- sqrt(mse)
ss_res <- sum((test_data$mpg - pred_mpg)^2)
```

(continued)

Chapter 5 (continued)

```
ss_tot <- sum((test_data$mpg - mean(test_data$mpg))^2)
rsq <- 1 - ss_res / ss_tot

# 9) Print metrics
print(paste("Test MSE:", round(mse, 2)))
print(paste("Test RMSE:", round(rmse, 2)))
print(paste("Test R-squared:", round(rsq, 2)))

# -------------------------------------
# Ridge Regression on mtcars with glmnet
# -------------------------------------

# Load required libraries
library(caret)
library(glmnet)

# Load the dataset
data(mtcars)

# Set random seed for reproducibility
set.seed(123)

# Split data: 80% training, 20% testing
trainIndex <- createDataPartition(mtcars$mpg, p = 0.8, list =
FALSE)
train_data <- mtcars[trainIndex, ]
test_data  <- mtcars[-trainIndex, ]

# Prepare predictor matrix and response vector
x_train <- as.matrix(train_data[, c('wt', 'hp', 'cyl')])
y_train <- train_data$mpg
x_test  <- as.matrix(test_data[, c('wt', 'hp', 'cyl')])
y_test  <- test_data$mpg

# Fit ridge regression model (alpha = 0)
ridge_model <- glmnet(x_train, y_train, alpha = 0)

# Predictions using the fitted model (alpha = 0)
pred_mpg <- predict(ridge_model, s = 0.1, newx = x_test)
```

(continued)

Chapter 5 (continued)

```
# Evaluation model performance
mse <- mean((y_test - pred_mpg)^2)
rmse <- sqrt(mse)
rsq <- 1 - sum((y_test - pred_mpg)^2) / sum((y_test - mean(y_test))
^2)

print(paste("Test MSE:", round(mse, 2)))
print(paste("Test RMSE:", round(rmse, 2)))
print(paste("Test R-squared:", round(rsq, 2)))

# ------------------------------------
# Lasso Regression on mtcars with glmnet
# ------------------------------------

# Load required libraries
library(caret)
library(glmnet)

# Load dataset
data(mtcars)

# Set random seed for reproducibility
set.seed(123)

# Split data into training and testing sets (80%-20%)
trainIndex <- createDataPartition(mtcars$mpg, p = 0.8, list =
FALSE)
train_data <- mtcars[trainIndex, ]
test_data  <- mtcars[-trainIndex, ]

# Prepare predictor matrices and response vectors
x_train <- as.matrix(train_data[, c("wt", "hp", "cyl")])
y_train <- train_data$mpg
x_test  <- as.matrix(test_data[, c("wt", "hp", "cyl")])
y_test  <- test_data$mpg

# Fit lasso regression model (alpha = 1 for lasso)
lasso_model <- glmnet(x_train, y_train, alpha = 1)
```

(continued)

Chapter 5 (continued)

```
# Select optimal lambda using cross-validation
cv_lasso <- cv.glmnet(x_train, y_train, alpha = 1)
best_lambda <- cv_lasso$lambda.min

# Make predictions on test data
pred_mpg <- predict(lasso_model, s = best_lambda, new = x_test)

# Evaluate model performance
mse <- mean((y_test - pred_mpg)^2)
rmse <- sqrt(mse)

print(paste("Test MSE:", round(mse, 2)))
print(paste("Test RMSE:", round(rmse, 2)))

# Generic Evaluation with MSE, RMSE and RSQ

# Example codes to evaluate regression models in R

# Assuming actual_mpg are true observed values, pred_mpg are model
predictions

# Mean Squared Error (MSE)
mse <- mean((actual_mpg - pred_mpg)^2)

# Root Mean Squared Error (RMSE)
rmse <- sqrt(mse)

# R-squared
rsq <- 1 - sum((actual_mpg - pred_mpg)^2) / sum((actual_mpg - mean
(actual_mpg))^2)

# Display the evaluation metrics
print(paste("Mean Squared Error (MSE):", round(mse, 2)))
print(paste("Root Mean Squared Error (RMSE):", round(rmse, 2)))
print(paste("R-squared:", round(rsq, 2)))
```

Chapter 6

```
# K-means clustering on iris (complete, reproducible example)

# Load required libraries
install.packages(c("ggplot2", "cluster","factoextra"))
library(ggplot2)
library(cluster)
library(factoextra)

# Load and prepare the dataset
data(iris)
iris_data <- scale(iris[, -5]) #Remove species label and scale
features

# Set seed for reproducibility
set.seed(123)

# Apply K-means clustering (3 clusters, as there are 3 iris species)
kmeans_result <- kmeans(iris_data, centers = 3, nstart = 25)

# Add cluster assignments to the original dataset
iris$Cluster <- as.factor(kmeans_result$cluster)

# Visualize clusters using fviz_cluster
fviz_cluster(kmeans_result, data = iris_data,
       geom = "point", ellipse.type = "norm",
       ggtheme = theme_minimal())

# Evaluate clustering performance using contingency table
table(iris$Species, iris$Cluster)

# Hierarchical clustering

# Libraries
# install.packages(c("cluster", "factoextra")) # if needed
library(cluster)
library(factoextra)

# Data and scaled_data
data("USArrests")
```

(continued)

Chapter 6 (continued)

```
data <- na.omit(USArrests)
scaled_data <- scale(data)

# Distance matrix
dist_matrix <- dist(scaled_data, method = "euclidean")

# Hierarchical clustering (complete linkage)
hc_complete <- hclust(dist_matrix, method = "complete")

# Dendrogram
plot(hc_complete,
   main = "USArrests — Hierarchical Clustering (complete
linkage)",
   xlab = "", sub = "", cex = 0.6)

# Rectangles to show k clusters
k <- 3
rect.hclust(hc_complete, k = k, border = "red")

# Cluster visualization with factoextra
clusters <- cutree(hc_complete, k = k)
fviz_cluster(
 list(data = scaled_data, cluster = clusters),
 main = sprintf("USArrests — Cluster Plot (k = %d)", k),
 ellipse.type = "t",
 repel = TRUE
)

# PCA
# Install if needed:
# install.packages("factoextra")

library(datasets)
library(factoextra)

# load data and scale
data("USArrests")
scaled_data <- scale(USArrests)
```

(continued)

Chapter 6 (continued)

```
# PCA
pca_result <- prcomp(scaled_data, center = FALSE, scale. = FALSE)

# variance explained (eigenvalues)
fviz_eig(pca_result, addlabels = TRUE, main = "USArrests — PCA:
Variance Explained")

# biplot
fviz_pca_biplot(
 pca_result,
 repel = TRUE,
 title = "USArrests — PCA Biplot (scaled)"
)
```

Chapter 7

```
# For reproducibility
set.seed(123)

n <- 100

age <- sample(20:60, n, replace = TRUE)
gender <- sample(c("Male", "Female"), n, replace = TRUE)
blood_pressure <- round(rnorm(n, mean = 120, sd = 15), 1)
risk <- ifelse((age > 45 & blood_pressure >= 130) | blood_pressure >
140 , "high", "low")

notes_samples <- c(
 "Patient reports chest pain and shortness of breath,",
 "Routine checkup. No significant complaints.",
 "Elevated blood pressure observed during visit.",
 "Patient advised to reduce salt intake.",
 "Reports frequent headaches and dizziness.",
 "No history of cardiovascular issues. Regular physical activity."
)
doctors_notes <- sample(notes_samples, n, replace = TRUE)
```

(continued)

Chapter 7 (continued)

```
df <- data.frame(
 age = age,
 gender = gender,
 blood_pressure = blood_pressure,
 risk = factor(risk, levels = c("low","high")),
 doctors_notes = doctors_notes,
 stringsAsFactors = FALSE
)

head(df, 10)

#SVM
library(e1071)

# Fit the SVM using age and blood_pressure as predictors
svm_model <- svm(risk ~ age + blood_pressure, data = df, kernel =
"linear")

# Predict on the same data (for a quick check)
pred <- predict(svm_model, newdata = df)

# Evaluate
accuracy <- mean(pred == df$risk)
print(accuracy)

# (Optional) Visualize the decision boundary if desired
library(ggplot2)
xrange <- seq(min(df$age), max(df$age), length= 100)
yrange <- seq(min(df$blood_pressure), max(df$blood_pressure),
length = 100)
grid <- expand.grid(age = xrange, blood_pressure = yrange)
grid$pred <- predict(svm_model, newdata = grid)
ggplot(df, aes(x = age, y = blood_pressure, color = risk)) +
 geom_point(size = 2) +
 geom_contour(data = grid, aes(z = as.numeric(pred)), breaks =
1.5, color = "black") +
 labs(title = "SVM Decision Boundary", x = "Age", y = "Blood
Pressure") +
 theme_minimal()
```

(continued)

Chapter 7 (continued)

```
# Gradient Boosting
# Load required packages

library(xgboost)
library(ggplot2)

# Prepare label (1 = High, 0 = Low)
df$label <- ifelse(df$risk == "High", 1L, 0L)

# Fit model
xgb_data <- xgb.DMatrix(data = as.matrix(df[, c("age",
"blood_pressure")]), label = df$label)
xgb_model <- xgboost(data = xgb_data, nrounds = 50, objective =
"binary:logistic", verbose = 0)

# Predict on the same data
pred_prob <- predict(xgb_model, as.matrix(df[, c("age",
"blood_pressure")]))
pred_class <- factor(ifelse(pred_prob > 0.5, "High", "Low"),
levels = levels(df$risk))

# Accuracy
accuracy <- mean(pred_class == df$risk)
print(paste("Accuracy:", round(accuracy, 3)))

ggplot(df, aes(x = age, y = blood_pressure, color = risk)) +
 geom_point(size = 2) +
 geom_contour(data = grid,
       aes(z = as.numeric(pred == "high")),
       breaks = 0.5,
       color = "blue") +
 labs(title = "Gradient Boosting Decision Boundary",
   x = "Age", y = "Blood Pressure") +
 theme_minimal()

# Neural network (nnet) — binary classification for risk
library(nnet)

# Prepare binary label: 1 = High, 0 = Low
df$label <- ifelse(df$risk == "High", 1, 0)
```

(continued)

Chapter 7 (continued)

```
# 2) Fit model (2 inputs -> hidden size 4 -> 1 output)
nn_model <- nnet(label ~ age + blood_pressure,
          data = df,
          size = 4, maxit = 500, trace = FALSE)

# 3) Predict probabilities and classes
nn_pred_prob <- as.numeric(predict(nn_model, df, type = "raw"))
nn_pred <- ifelse(nn_pred_prob > 0.5, "High", "Low")

# 4) Accuracy
accuracy <- mean(nn_pred == df$risk)
print(paste("Accuracy:", round(accuracy, 3)))

# 5) Visualization of decision regions
library(ggplot2)

xrange <- seq(min(df$age, na.rm = TRUE), max(df$age, na.rm =
TRUE), length.out = 200)
yrange <- seq(min(df$blood_pressure, na.rm = TRUE), max
(df$blood_pressure, na.rm = TRUE), length.out = 200)
grid <- expand.grid(age = xrange, blood_pressure = yrange)

grid$pred_prob <- as.numeric(predict(nn_model, grid, type =
"raw"))

ggplot(df, aes(x = age, y = blood_pressure, color = risk)) +
 geom_point(size = 2) +
 labs(title = "Neural Network Decision Boundary",
    x = "Age", y = "Blood Pressure") +
 theme_minimal()

# NLP
# Install required packages if not already installed
if (!require(tm)) install.packages("tm")
if (!require(wordcloud)) install.packages("wordcloud")
if (!require(RColorBrewer)) install.packages("RColorBrewer")
library(tm)
library(wordcloud)
library(RColorBrewer)
```

(continued)

Chapter 7 (continued)

```
# Assume your data frame is df with a column `doctors_notes`
# Step 1: Create a text corpus
corpus <- Corpus(VectorSource(df$doctors_notes))

# Step 2: Clean the text
corpus <- tm_map(corpus, content_transformer(tolower))
corpus <- tm_map(corpus, removePunctuation)
corpus <- tm_map(corpus, removeNumbers)
corpus <- tm_map(corpus, removeWords, stopwords("en"))
corpus <- tm_map(corpus, stripWhitespace)

# Step 3: Create a document-term matrix
dtm <- TermDocumentMatrix(corpus)
m <- as.matrix(dtm)

# Step 4: Calculate word frequencies
word_freqs <- sort(rowSums(m), decreasing = TRUE)

# Step 5: Display the top 10 most common words
print(head(word_freqs, 10))

# Step 6: Visualize with a word cloud
set.seed(123) # For reproducibility
wordcloud(words = names(word_freqs),
 freq = word_freqs,
 min.freq = 1,
 scale = c(3, 0.5),
 colors = brewer.pal(8, "Dark2"),
 random.order = FALSE)
```

Chapter 8

```
# Load required libraries
library(caret)
library(dplyr)
library(readr)

# Set seed for reproducibility
set.seed(123)
```

(continued)

Chapter 8 (continued)

```
# Load the dataset
data <- read_csv("simulated_ehr_dataset.csv")

# Convert appropriate variables to factors
categorical_vars <- c("Gender", "Income_Level",
"Smoking_Status", "Exercise_Level", "SUD_Status")
data[categorical_vars] <- lapply(data[categorical_vars], as.
factor)

# Stratified train-test split (80/20)
trainIndex <- createDataPartition(data$SUD_Status, p = 0.8, list
= FALSE)
train <- data[trainIndex, ]
test <- data[-trainIndex, ]

# Identify numeric columns for scaling
numeric_vars <- c("Age", "BMI", "Systolic_BP", "Diastolic_BP",
"Glucose", "Mental_Health_Score", "Family_History_SUD")

# Apply standard scaling (Z-score normalization)
preProcValues <- preProcess(train[, numeric_vars], method = c
("center", "scale"))

train_scaled <- train
train_scaled[, numeric_vars] <- predict(preProcValues, train[,
numeric_vars])

test_scaled <- test
test_scaled[, numeric_vars] <- predict(preProcValues, test[,
numeric_vars])

# Check result
str(train_scaled)
str(test_scaled)

# Load required libraries
library(caret)
library(dplyr)
```

(continued)

Chapter 8 (continued)

```
# Set seed for reproducibility
set.seed(123)

# Ensure SUD_Status is a factor
train$SUD_Status <- as.factor(train$SUD_Status)
test$SUD_Status <- as.factor(test$SUD_Status)

# Run logistic regression using all predictors
logit_model <- glm(SUD_Status ~ ., data = train, family = binomial)

# Display model coefficients
summary(logit_model)

# Predict on test data (probability output)
pred_probs <- predict(logit_model, newdata = test, type =
"response")

# Convert probabilities to class labels (threshold = 0.5)
pred_labels <- ifelse(pred_probs > 0.5, 1, 0)
pred_labels <- as.factor(pred_labels)

# Confusion matrix
confusionMatrix(pred_labels, test$SUD_Status, positive = "1")

# Load necessary libraries
library(rpart)
library(rpart.plot)
library(caret)

# Set seed for reproducibility
set.seed(123)

# Ensure the target variable is a factor
train$SUD_Status <- as.factor(train$SUD_Status)
test$SUD_Status <- as.factor(test$SUD_Status)

# Train the decision tree with max depth = 4
tree_model2 <- rpart(SUD_Status ~ .,
          data = train,
```

(continued)

Chapter 8 (continued)

```
          method = "class",
          control = rpart.control(maxdepth = 4))

# Visualize the tree
rpart.plot(tree_model2,
      type = 3,
      extra = 104,
      cex = 1,
      tweak = 0.7,
      compress = TRUE,
      box.palette = "BuGn",
      fallen.leaves = TRUE)

# Generate predictions on test data
tree_predictions <- predict(tree_model2, newdata = test, type =
"class")

# Evaluate model performance using confusion matrix
confusionMatrix(tree_predictions, test$SUD_Status, positive =
"1")

# Load required libraries
library(randomForest)
library(caret)

# Set seed for reproducibility
set.seed(123)

# Ensure the outcome variable is a factor
train$SUD_Status <- as.factor(train$SUD_Status)
test$SUD_Status <- as.factor(test$SUD_Status)

# Train the random forest model using all predictors
rf_model <- randomForest(SUD_Status ~ ., data = train, ntree =
500, importance = TRUE)

# Generate predictions on the test set
rf_pred <- predict(rf_model, newdata = test)
```

(continued)

Chapter 8 (continued)

```
# Convert predictions to binary levels (0 or 1) if needed
# (This step is included for consistency; rf_pred is already a
factor with levels 0 and 1)
rf_pred_binary <- ifelse(rf_pred == "1", 1, 0)
rf_pred_binary <- as.factor(rf_pred_binary)

# Evaluate performance using a confusion matrix
confusionMatrix(rf_pred_binary, test$SUD_Status, positive =
"1")

importance(rf_model)

varImpPlot(rf_model)

plot(rf_model)

################################
##############################
## 1. Setup
#################################
#############################
library(caret)       # data splitting & performance
library(rpart)       # decision tree
library(rpart.plot)  # (optional) tree plot
library(randomForest) # random forest
library(pROC)        # AUC / ROC curves

set.seed(123)        # reproducibility

##################################
############################
## 2. Read data & stratified split (80/20)
###################################
###########################
data <- read.csv("simulated_ehr_dataset.csv")

# ensure target is factor
data$SUD_Status <- as.factor(data$SUD_Status)
```

(continued)

Chapter 8 (continued)

```
idx <- createDataPartition(data$SUD_Status, p = 0.8, list =
FALSE)
train <- data[idx, ]
test <- data[-idx, ]

####################################
##########################
## 3. Fit three models
#####################################
#########################
#--- (a) Logistic regression --------------------------------
logit_mod <- glm(SUD_Status ~ ., data = train, family = binomial)

#--- (b) Decision tree (depth capped at 4) ------------------
tree_mod <- rpart(
 SUD_Status ~ ., data = train, method = "class",
 control = rpart.control(maxdepth = 4)
)

#--- (c) Random forest --------------------------------------
rf_mod  <- randomForest(SUD_Status ~ ., data = train,
             ntree = 500, importance = TRUE)

######################################
########################
## 4. Generate predictions & probabilities
#######################################
#######################
# Positive class is "1"
# Logistic
logit_prob <- predict(logit_mod, newdata = test, type =
"response")
logit_pred <- factor(ifelse(logit_prob > 0.5, 1, 0), levels = c
(0,1))

# Decision tree
tree_prob <- predict(tree_mod, newdata = test, type = "prob")[,
"1"]
tree_pred <- predict(tree_mod, newdata = test, type = "class")
```

(continued)

Chapter 8 (continued)

```
# Random forest
rf_prob  <- predict(rf_mod, newdata = test, type = "prob")[, "1"]
rf_pred  <- predict(rf_mod, newdata = test)  # already factor 0/1

########################################
#####################
## 5. Evaluate each model
#########################################
####################
eval_metrics <- function(truth, pred, prob) {
 cm <- confusionMatrix(pred, truth, positive = "1")
 data.frame(
  Accuracy  = cm$overall["Accuracy"],
  Sens    = cm$byClass["Sensitivity"],
  Spec    = cm$byClass["Specificity"],
  BalAcc   = cm$byClass["Balanced Accuracy"],
  AUC     = auc(truth, prob)[1]
 )
}

results <- rbind(
 Logistic    = eval_metrics(test$SUD_Status, logit_pred,
logit_prob),
 DecisionTree = eval_metrics(test$SUD_Status, tree_pred,
tree_prob),
 RandomForest = eval_metrics(test$SUD_Status, rf_pred,
rf_prob)
)

#############################################################
## 6. Display comparison table
#############################################################
print(round(results, 4))

#############################################################
## 7. (Optional) plot ROC curves on same graph
#############################################################
plot(roc(test$SUD_Status, logit_prob), col = "black", lwd =
2, main = "ROC Comparison")
plot(roc(test$SUD_Status, tree_prob), col = "blue", lwd = 2, add
```

(continued)

Chapter 8 (continued)

```
= TRUE)
plot(roc(test$SUD_Status, rf_prob),  col = "green", lwd = 2, add =
TRUE)
legend("bottomright",
    legend = c("Logistic", "Decision Tree", "Random Forest"),
    col   = c("black", "blue", "green"), lwd = 2)

##############################################################
# End of script
##############################################################
```

Chapter 9

```
#                ----------------                   Packages
--------------------------------------------------
if (!requireNamespace("lime", quietly = TRUE)) install.packages
("lime")
if (!requireNamespace("caret", quietly = TRUE)) install.packages
("caret")
if (!requireNamespace("randomForest", quietly = TRUE)) install.
packages("randomForest")
if (!requireNamespace("dplyr", quietly = TRUE)) install.packages
("dplyr")

# ---------------- Load required packages ----------------
library(caret)
library(randomForest)
library(lime)
library(dplyr)
library(ggplot2)

# ---------------- Prepare the data ----------------
# Ensure target variable is a factor for classification
train$SUD_Status <- as.factor(train$SUD_Status)
test$SUD_Status  <- as.factor(test$SUD_Status)
```

(continued)

Chapter 9 (continued)

```
# Split into predictors and outcome
train_x <- train %>% select(-SUD_Status)
train_y <- train$SUD_Status

# --------------- Train the model using caret ---------------
set.seed(123)
rf_model2 <- train(
 x = train_x,
 y = train_y,
 method = "rf",
 ntree = 500,
 trControl = trainControl(method = "cv", number = 5)
)

# --------------- Build LIME explainer
-----------------------------------
explainer <- lime::lime(
 x          = train_x,      # predictor variables from training data
 model      = rf_model2,    # trained caret model
 bin_continuous = TRUE,     # discretize numeric variables
 n_bins     = 5,            # number of bins for binning
 quantile_bins = TRUE       # use quantile-based binning
)

# ==========================================
==================================
# 📊 Part 1: Generic feature importance from 100 test cases
# ==================================
==========================================
set.seed(42)
sample_size <- 100 # number of cases to use for generic explanation
cases_x <- test %>%
 dplyr::slice_sample(n = sample_size) %>%
 dplyr::select(-SUD_Status) # keep only predictor variables

# Generate LIME explanations for the sample
explanations <- lime::explain(
```

(continued)

Chapter 9 (continued)

```
 x          = cases_x,
 explainer   = explainer,
 n_labels    = 1,          # explain the top predicted class
 n_features  = 8,          # number of features to include per case
 n_samples   = 5000,
 dist_fun    = "gower",
 kernel_width = 0.75
)

# Aggregate feature importance
generic_importance <- explanations %>%
 dplyr::group_by(feature) %>%
 dplyr::summarise(mean_abs_weight = mean(abs(feature_weight)))
%>%
 dplyr::arrange(desc(mean_abs_weight))

print(generic_importance)

# Plot aggregated importance
ggplot(generic_importance,
    aes(x = reorder(feature, mean_abs_weight),
       y = mean_abs_weight)) +
 geom_col(fill = "steelblue") +
 coord_flip() +
 labs(
  title = "Average Absolute LIME Feature Importance (n =
100 cases)",
  x = "Feature",
  y = "Average |Weight|"
 )

# ==================================================
================================
```

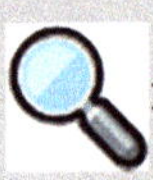

```
# Part 2: Explain one specific observation
# =============================================
=====================================
# Select one high-risk case (SUD_Status == 1)
case_1_idx <- which(test$SUD_Status == 1)[1]
case_1_x <- test[case_1_idx, ] %>% select(-SUD_Status)
```

(continued)

Chapter 9 (continued)

```
# Generate LIME explanation
explanation_1 <- lime::explain(
 x         = case_1_x,
 explainer    = explainer,
 n_labels    = 1,
 n_features   = 8,
 n_samples    = 5000,
 dist_fun    = "gower",
 kernel_width = 0.75
)

# Plot LIME explanation for one case
plot_features(explanation_1)

# ========================================
========================================
# 🔍 Part 3: Explain six observations and visualize together
# ========================================
========================================
# Select six positive-class observations
case_6_idx <- which(test$SUD_Status == 1)[1:6]
cases_6_x <- test[case_6_idx, ] %>% select(-SUD_Status)

# Generate explanations for six cases
explanation_6 <- lime::explain(
 x         = cases_6_x,
 explainer    = explainer,
 n_labels    = 1,
 n_features   = 8,
 n_samples    = 5000,
 dist_fun    = "gower",
 kernel_width = 0.75
)

# Plot all six explanations in one faceted plot (3 columns,
automatic rows)
plot_features(
 explanation_6,
 ncol = 3
)
```

Index

R. Leung, *Leveraging GenAI for Machine Learning Education in Public Health*,
https://doi.org/10.1007/978-3-032-08677-8

MIX
Papier aus verantwortungsvollen Quellen
Paper from responsible sources
FSC® C105338

If you have any concerns about our products,
you can contact us on
ProductSafety@springernature.com

In case Publisher is established outside the EU,
the EU authorized representative is:
Springer Nature Customer Service Center GmbH
Europaplatz 3, 69115 Heidelberg, Germany

Printed by Libri Plureos GmbH
in Hamburg, Germany